Kitchen Cures

Homemade
Remedies
for
Your Health

Reader's Digest

New York | Montreal

Library of Congress Cataloging in Publication Data is available upon request.

ISBN 13: 978-1-62145-386-4 (hardcover)
       978-1-62145-477-9 (paperback)

We are committed to both the quality of our products and the service we provide to our customers. We value your comments, so please feel free to contact us.

> Reader's Digest Adult Trade Publishing
> 44 South Broadway
> White Plains, NY 10601

For more Reader's Digest products and information, visit our website:
> www.rd.com (in the United States)
> www.readersdigest.ca (in Canada)

Printed in China

10 9 8 7 6 5 4 3 2 1

NOTE TO READERS
The information in this book should not be substituted for, or used to alter, medical therapy without your doctor's advice. For a specific health problem, consult your physician for guidance. The mention of any products, retail businesses, or websites in this book does not imply or constitute an endorsement by the authors or by Trusted Media Brands, Inc.

Cures That Work

The proof is in! Home remedies often rival or even exceed the healing power of drugstore medicines. Recent studies have shown that . . .

Aloe gel improves psoriasis better than prescription cream

Baking soda slows the progress of chronic kidney disease

Clove oil is a powerful fungus killer

Green tea can help you lose weight

Chamomile is not just a soothing tea

Honey truly does enhance wound healing

Smelling lavender and rosemary oil reduces anxiety

And that's just a taste! *Kitchen Cures* is your comprehensive guide to natural healing at home. Here are hundreds of remedies for the most common health ailments and conditions. Save money, save time, heal faster and safer . . . just turn the page!

contents

{ PART FOUR }

practical home healing 232

Tips and lists to help you get started

index 247

folk healing the modern way

Welcome to a whole new world of natural home rememdies

When grandparents reminisce about the good ol' days, they probably don't talk much about how clever they were at remedying things like colds, scrapes, or toothaches. But for thousands of years, the majority of healing was pretty much a do-it-yourself enterprise. Except for serious emergencies, everyone needed to have at least a smattering of healing ability to preserve and protect their family's health.

That meant learning to heal with whatever staples they had on hand. And, strange as some of those old cures sound today (imagine plastering your chest with mustard paste), it turns out that our forebears knew what they were doing. Home remedies really did work, and still do.

So why are they used so infrequently today? Over time, as researchers discovered effective new drugs, treatments and "procedures" for remedying diseases and injuries, we lost the need—and the know-how and confidence—for using home remedies to treat common health problems. Instead, we've come to rely much more heavily on pills, doctors, and store-bought cures for all that ails us.

But times are changing again. In laboratories around the world, researchers in recent years have explored and confirmed the healing power of many of our favorite pantry items. In these costly and complicated times, it's just good common sense to rediscover time-honored home remedies for treating simple but annoying woes—before you pay for an expensive doctor's visit.

Inexpensive health solutions

This book provides hundreds of ways to cure yourself and your family safely and inexpensively. Got athlete's foot? Instead of losing half a day seeing a doctor, and then writing a check for an expensive antifungal lotion, you can try a homemade tea-tree oil remedy for just pennies. Got a hacking cough? A tea made from your supply of dried thyme may clear it up in a day or two, without the need for a prescription drug or an over-the-counter cough syrup—which research has recently shown, doesn't work very well, if at all.

That said, not every remedy in this book will work for everyone. That's true for store-bought medicine, and it's true for homemade remedies. But unlike some prescription drugs, these simple, natural recipes are less likely to cost you significant money or to have unpleasant side effects.

Consider the satisfaction you'll derive from learning how to make delicious, soothing teas from herbs and spices you probably already have in your pantry. You'll discover healing creams and ointments you can whip up from ingredients like olive oil and honey, and digestive aids that require nothing more than a little baking soda, a bit of ginger, or a dash of hot sauce. No matter what minor ills or accidents befall your family members, just turn to the index where you'll find a cheap, effective, easy-to-make remedy to fix them right up.

Remedies worth sharing

In compiling this collection, we reached back through time to find the most effective, time-tested home remedies we could get our hands on. We discovered herbal recipes from traditional Chinese and Indian medicine. We unearthed healing wisdom, born of necessity, that Native Americans and North American pioneers handed down from generation to generation. We sorted through books on regional folk medicine from all over Europe, South America, and beyond. Our search for these remedies carried us through history, from the era of Hippocrates to the battlefields of World War I to the backyard gardens of 21st century herbal healers.

Though we cast a wide net, our final criteria for the best home remedies were determined using a highly selective process.

• First, remedies had to come from common ingredients found in kitchen pantries. Occasionally, we stretched our notion of "pantry" a bit to accommodate a few refrigerated items (eggs and yogurt, for example) or the aloe plant, which you can grow on a windowsill.

• Second, remedies had to be simple to whip up and easy to use. And naturally, they all had to be safe. We put the remedies to a test: Is this something we might actually use ourselves? Or would recommend to a loved one? Or use on our own children? They made the cut when we could answer, "Yes, these are remedies we would absolutely use."

• Third, the remedies had to stand the test of time. For example, when we saw an herb that was used to treat nervous conditions from the time of the Romans to the 19th century, we knew we were on to something. We then searched the scientific literature to make sure that there was a medical rationale for its effectiveness and safety.

One thing home remedies have going for them is that they harness the power of ritual—in itself a potent healing tool. The very act of making a remedy from scratch, applying it with love, and believing that it will help your loved one get better has healing powers that may enhance or even trump ingredients in the "cure." So we've often included time-tested remedies that combine safe, gentle, healing ingredients and a soothing application, even if they haven't been scientifically proven.

After we rejected all the odd, less-credible, more-complicated, and slightly risky remedies, what remained were the wonderful (and sometimes wondrous) remedies you'll find in this book—hundreds that have helped heal millions of people over hundreds, if not thousands, of years. Finally, every single one of these remedies was carefully vetted by our medical reviewer to ensure that all are safe for you to use as recommended.

Use kitchen cures wisely

If traditional cures were used daily for thousands of years, they probably work or else people wouldn't have used them. But there are always risks—of side effects, of interactions with drugs, or of simply being the wrong remedy. The home remedies in this book are supported by strong anecdotal evidence of their effectiveness—and in many cases by scientific studies—and they have been carefully screened for safety by our medical advisor. But there are times when you'll want to exercise extra caution, such as:

If you are pregnant. Do not take any herbs, supplements, or over-the-counter medications without first checking with your doctor. Even innocuous remedies might have unwanted effects on your pregnancy or your baby.

If you are taking prescription medication. Talk to your doctor about possible interactions between your prescribed medication and any remedies recommended in this book. And tell your doctor about any other supplements or medications that you take at the same time—particularly if you have a chronic condition such as diabetes or heart disease.

If you know you are allergic to a food or medication. Exercise caution or consult your doctor before you eat or drink any remedy that might contain the allergen.

If you have a serious health condition. Pay special attention to "When to Call the Doctor" at the beginning of each chapter. The purpose of these home remedies is to help you deal with everyday ailments and improve your overall health—not to mask serious conditions that require medical treatment.

If you are treating a child or infant. Some home remedies just aren't appropriate for children or babies. Unless a remedy is specifically recommended for children, ask your pediatrician for advice before treating your kids.

If you are experiencing unwanted effects. Although side effects from using safe home remedies are uncommon, allergic reactions can occur, even if you've never been allergic to something before. If you have a reaction, immediately stop using the product.

When using essential oils. These products are highly concentrated natural chemicals, and so pose some risks. Most essential oils must be diluted in carrier oil before being applied to the skin. Some oils, particularly citrus ones, can make your skin extra-sensitive to the sun, and should be applied with caution or not at all before sun exposure. Never swallow or even taste essential oils; most are toxic when taken internally. Keep bottles and jars sealed and out of the reach of children. Finally, if an essential oil is accidentally swallowed, do not induce vomiting. Call a poison hotline or get the person to an emergency room immediately.

Winning combinations

No matter how much we believe in home remedies, few of us are willing to completely turn our backs on conventional medicine. What most of us want is the best of both worlds—the cutting-edge tools of modern medicine combined with the natural, at-home treatments that earlier generations depended on. As more than one expert has noted, if you get hit by a car, or have a heart attack or stroke, you want the best, newest, state-of-the-art treatments medical science has to offer. But if you have a chronic condition, such as diabetes, arthritis, or irritable bowel syndrome, you might want treatments that blend natural remedies with the latest up-to-date methods.

This approach, known as integrative medicine, makes wonderful sense. If you have heart disease or diabetes, for example, you want the most advanced care available. Yet there's so much you can do yourself at the same time—not only to relieve symptoms and feel better, but also to give nature a hand and help your body recover more quickly or even reverse the condition. Be sure to let your doctor know that you're interested in using as many natural approaches as makes sense for your condition.

It might surprise you to hear your endocrinologist suggest, for example, that you switch breakfast cereals. That's because she's seen the studies that suggest cinnamon can help lower your blood-sugar levels. And your cardiologist might have a positive take on herbs like garlic, which is proven to help reduce blood pressure and lower cholesterol.

One thing about home remedies is that they are often more art than science. Many of the traditional formulas we found for teas, creams, steams and baths called for measurements that, truth be told, weren't well defined. For instance, a grandmother may have written, a "spoonful" of honey, a "handful" of garlic, or a "few pinches" of baking soda. Happily, in many cases the exact amounts aren't critical to the remedy's effectiveness. Still, for best results, follow the recipes as written. We've edited them to include ingredients most likely to provide some direct health benefits, while omitting those that are ineffective, hard to come by, or likely to cause problems.

Few of the remedies in this book require special supplies—just the diverse items you'll find on the shelves in your kitchen cabinets. Occasionally, we'll include ingredients you probably don't have (such as beeswax), which are easy to find and are essential to some very useful remedies.

Temporary relief, or even a cure, may be just a few steps away. If one remedy doesn't work for you, try another. If it does work, be sure to tell a loved one or friend so that they might one day benefit from it, too.

Happy healing!

top pantry healers

An A-to-Z guide to the natural medicines sitting on your kitchen shelves

You probably don't look inside your kitchen cabinet and think *drugstore*. But for untold generations, that's exactly the role kitchen pantries have performed. You'd be surprised how many everyday staples have a successful second career as natural medicine. After all, it's a lot quicker, simpler, and cheaper to make a paste of baking soda and water and dab it on a bug bite than it is to drive to the drugstore for an expensive anti-itch cream.

In the pages ahead, you'll discover the remarkable healing benefits of many familiar, inexpensive items that are already sitting right there on your pantry shelves. You'll learn how to harness the healing power of time-tested staples like honey, vinegar, baking soda, and plain old salt. The antinausea power of ginger. The heart protection of canned salmon and sardines. Mustard's unique ability to treat lung problems, and turmeric's potential for preventing serious chronic diseases—and even cancer.

And don't miss the special features posted in each entry, including shopping tips, safety information, and indispensable advice about how to buy and store your pantry healing ingredients to retain their maximum potency and effectiveness.

aloe

Aloe is one of the most versatile kitchen healers around—but please don't keep this one in your pantry. Instead, you'll want to grow the spiny succulent plant on your windowsill, because its stalky leaves contain a gel-like substance that healers think of as Mother Nature's first aid kit. This lily cousin thrives on neglect and is so hardy that you'll be able to harvest its wound-repairing, skin-moisturizing, ulcer-soothing magic for years to come.

rooted in history

Aloe (*Aloe vera* and *Aloe barbadensis*) has been used medicinally for at least 5,500 years. The first documentation of its healing uses are on an Egyptian papyrus dating back to 3500 BC. Legend has it that Aristotle convinced Alexander the Great to invade the island of Socotra in the Indian Ocean just for its aloe supply, which healed his warriors' wounds and got them back on the battlefield faster. In a very different use, Cleopatra—and other gorgeous leading ladies of history—reportedly relied on aloe for beautifying their complexions.

Aloe plants migrated from Africa to America in the 17th and 18th centuries, where they were soon adopted by healers in the New World.

what's in it?

Though aloe is 99 percent water, the clear gel inside the leaves contains a handy assortment of potent healing compounds. Take glycoproteins and polysaccharides, for example. Glycoproteins speed healing by stopping pain and inflammation. Polysaccharides moisturize skin, stimulate its growth and repair, and enhance wound healing. What's more, aloe gel contains a pain-relieving substance called bradykininase that helps reduce swelling. The mineral magnesium lactate, another aloe gel component, soothes itching and eases allergic rashes.

what science says

In 2009, Iranian researchers reviewed 40 studies published about aloe's effectiveness as a skin treatment. They reported that there is scientific evidence to back using aloe gel for treating genital herpes, psoriasis, human papillomavirus, seborrheic dermatitis, frostbite, and burns.

The same year, a different team of Iranian scientists examined aloe's ability to heal second-degree skin burns. (Second-degree burns affect both the top and the second layers of the skin, causing painful blisters and inflammation.) The researchers compared aloe to a tried-and-true burn ointment called silver sulfadiazine, which prevents infection of second- and third-degree burns. As it turns out, the burns treated with aloe healed three days faster than those receiving the more standard medicine.

And in Thailand, researchers studying psoriasis treatments published a study that compared aloe to a conventional steroid cream. Eighty people with mild to moderate psoriasis were randomly treated with aloe vera or the steroid cream for eight weeks. The results were about the same, though the aloe treatment had a slight edge over the steroid treatment.

on the horizon

The same compounds that make aloe a smart treatment for skin problems intrigue scientists focused on finding solutions for problems like colitis and ulcers. As their thinking goes, if aloe can heal external wounds, it might just heal internal wounds. Turns out, they could be right. Studies conducted in the mid-1990s suggest that drinking pure aloe gel may help ease ulcerative colitis by reducing inflammation in the GI tract.

Good to Know

Aloe plants produce another substance called aloe latex, which comes from the skin of the aloe leaf. It's a bitter yellow liquid that performs as a powerful laxative. Too powerful, in fact. Classified as a stimulant laxative, it can cause severe cramping and diarrhea and can even affect your electrolytes, minerals that play a critical role in the body. Trust us, this is not good medicine for irregularity or constipation.

Aloe gel contains a pain-relieving substance that helps reduce swelling.

In one United Kingdom study, 44 people with ulcerative colitis were either given about 3 ounces of aloe vera gel twice a day or a sham juice for a month. Of the 30 people who took aloe, 9 people experienced symptom relief, compared to 1 person in the group of 14 people who took the fake treatment. The researchers noted that aloe was a safe treatment that needs more study.

Korean researchers put aloe to the test on rats with stomach ulcers and observed that taking aloe seemed to regenerate tissue cells. However, what works on a rat might not work on a human, so these results need confirmation via clinical trials conducted on people.

Finally, back in 2003, leading researchers from Harvard Medical School reviewed 109 studies that tested supplements for helping people control their blood sugar. They concluded that the results for aloe studies were promising but preliminary. Discuss aloe with your doctor if you're taking medications to lower your blood sugar.

BUYER's tip

The best aloe gel comes directly from a living plant. Just chop off a nice, thick stalk, slice it lengthwise, and squeeze the gel directly onto your skin. Be sure not to get the goo on your clothes; it will leave an ugly stain. You can find aloe plants at most places live plants are sold. They respond very well to almost no attention and grow nicely on a sunny windowsill.

No aloe plant? No problem. You can find pure aloe gel at most health food stores. Just read the label carefully to make sure the product is 100 percent pure aloe gel with no additional ingredients.

baking soda

Baking soda is without question the hardest working multitasker on your pantry shelf. It's an essential baking ingredient—it's what makes cakes, cookies, and other treats rise. It's also an effective and "green" household cleaner and a deodorizer that de-stinks cat pans, garbage cans, refrigerator interiors, and other smelly things—even feet and underarms. And as it turns out, baking soda is also a gentle, fast-acting remedy for a plethora of annoying health conditions, from diaper rash to sunburn pain.

what's in it?

Baking soda is a mildly alkaline salt that reacts easily with acids, releasing carbon dioxide and creating effervescence. Most baking soda—that is, sodium bicarbonate—is derived from soda ash that occurs naturally as an ore called trona. Trona is mined in the Green River Basin in Wyoming.

what science says

Good old-fashioned baking soda has recently captured the attention of kidney disease researchers. This cheap pantry item may slow the decline of kidney function in some people who have advanced chronic kidney disease. When people with advanced kidney disease took a small daily dose of baking soda in addition to their usual care, kidney function declined about two-thirds slower than it did in patients who didn't take baking soda. Kidney disease

USE FOR

Anal itching

Asthma

Athlete's foot

Bad breath

Bladder infections

Body odor

Canker sores

Diaper rash

Flatulence

Foot and
  underarm odor

Healthy teeth

Heartburn

Hives

Indigestion

Poison ivy/oak

Sore throat

Stings and bites

Sunburn

Good to Know

Baking soda meets standards as a safe food additive and can be used freely, with two critical caveats. First, anyone on a sodium-restricted diet should consult a physician before taking it internally, because it could increase sodium levels. Second, because baking soda contains sodium, don't use it regularly if you have high blood pressure or heart failure.

progressed rapidly in just 9 percent of people who took baking soda, compared to 45 percent of people who didn't take it. The people taking baking soda were also less likely to develop end-stage renal disease, a life-threatening condition that causes people to require dialysis. However, critics of the 2009 study take its results with a grain of salt. Here's why: The treatment wasn't compared to a placebo, and the researchers knew which patients were getting the baking soda and which weren't.

neutralize acid, soothe the itch

Baking soda's ability to take the itch and sting out of a variety of skin problems comes from its alkaline nature. Chemicals with pH values of 6 and lower are acids. Those with a pH of 8 or above are alkaline. (Water, which comes in at 7, is neutral.) With a pH of 9, baking soda is alkaline enough to take the edge off potentially harsh acids. This is how it eases heartburn, by neutralizing the stomach acid (hydrochloric acid) that causes heartburn's uncomfortable burning sensation.

That action also comes into play for relieving the itch and sting of bug bites, poison ivy, and poison oak. The same holds true for diaper rash: Baking soda lessens itching and helps irritated skin heal more quickly.

a box full of healing

Because baking soda lowers the bacteria-friendly acidic environment inside the bladder, it can be a useful home remedy for easing the discomfort of bladder infections. As a gargle for sore throats, it reduces pain-causing acids, and mixed with a little water as a tooth polish, it whitens teeth and combats the acids that gnaw away at tooth enamel. And it has the advantage of being less abrasive than most toothpaste. The baking soda paste will also help fight acne: Rubbing a blackhead gently with the paste for two to three minutes will loosen it. A dusting of baking soda under the arms or on the feet serves as an inexpensive deodorant.

cayenne pepper

People who don't like spicy foods often think that hot-pepper lovers are savaging their mouths and digestive systems. But nothing could be further from the truth. That burning sensation in your mouth when you eat foods spiced with cayenne pepper (*Capsicum annuum*) and its many hot-pepper cousins comes from capsaicin, the oily compound responsible for its many health benefits. Turns out that eating spicy foods does wonders for you—everything from managing pain to opening up clogged airways to potentially even managing diabetes.

what's in it?

The hotter a chili pepper is, the more capsaicin it contains. Capsaicin short-circuits pain by depleting nerve cells of a chemical called substance P, which helps transfer pain signals along nerve endings to the brain. Because of that pain-depleting action, you'll find capsaicin in many prescription and over-the-counter creams, ointments, and patches for arthritis and muscle pain. It's also used for treating postsurgical pain, shingles pain, and diabetes-related nerve pain.

But that's not all. Capsaicin also is a metabolism booster, speeding up your calorie-burning furnace for a couple of hours after eating. Plus hot peppers work as an anti-inflammatory. Finally, hot peppers contain plenty of vitamins A and C along with flavonoids and carotenoids, plant pigments that act as antioxidants.

USE FOR

Arthritis

Carpal tunnel syndrome

Colds and flu

Fever

Foot problems

Laryngitis

Nasal congestion

Nausea and vomiting

Nosebleed

Pain relief

Shingles

Sore throat

Toothache

Weight management

Cayenne pepper is available in the spice section at the supermarket. It is also known as ground red pepper.

Fresh cayenne peppers can burn or irritate skin. Wear rubber gloves when handling fresh hot peppers, don't touch your eyes or nose, and wash hands after preparing them. Same goes for the spice—use a utensil to measure and add to recipes, not your fingers. If you use topical capsaicin creams, be sure to follow label directions.

Good to Know

Because cayenne shrinks blood vessels in your nose and throat, it helps relieve congestion when you sprinkle some into hot soup. Or shake in as much as you can tolerate of hot sauce or other fiery condiments for the same congestion-busting effects.

rooted in history

All these benefits of cayenne pepper—not to mention the wonderful flavor it can add to our food—have been well known for a *very* long time. There's evidence that Native Americans have used cayenne as both a food and a medicine for at least 9,000 years. Traditional healers in India, China, Japan, and Korea use it to remedy digestive problems, poor appetite, and circulatory problems.

what science says

In one study, published in the *American Journal of Clinical Nutrition*, researchers found that people with diabetes who ate a meal laced liberally with chili pepper needed less insulin after eating to reduce their blood sugar, suggesting the spice may have antidiabetes benefits. Those results were backed by Thai researchers in 2009. Trouble is, you have to use at least a teaspoon of the stuff before you get the glucose-lowering benefit—which might be too much heat for people whose palates aren't fireproof.

on the horizon

Researchers are hard at work in labs all over the world, trying to figure out how to harness capsaicin's tumor-busting potential. At the Massachusetts Institute of Technology, scientists are studying capsaicin's effects on colon cancer cells. In a recent study, they learned that capsaicin can make cancer cells self-destruct because it affects levels of nitric oxide. Meanwhile, at Cedars-Sinai Medical Center at UCLA School of Medicine, scientists looked at capsaicin's effect on breast cancer cells. In a new study, they revealed that capsaicin slowed breast cancer cell growth in test tube models. In their animal studies, they reported that capsaicin decreased experimentally induced tumors in mice by 50 percent and inhibited the development of precancerous lesions by up to 80 percent.

Finally, in lab tests published in 2009, Taiwanese researchers showed that capsaicin makes stomach cancer cells self-destruct. It will likely take years of research before we know whether or not eating cayenne can prevent or treat cancer in humans. However, there's certainly no downside to eating the hot stuff regularly just in case.

chamomile

When the day has frazzled your nerves to the extent that you feel like pulling your hair out, it's time to sit down and have a nice cup of chamomile tea. And your nerves aren't the only thing chamomile tea is good at soothing: This herb is wonderful for easing digestive distress, skin irritations, and occasional mild insomnia.

rooted in history

Chamomile (*Matricaria recutita*) tea is made from the tiny daisy-like flowers of a lacy-leafed plant that now grows all over the world. This delicate, apple-scented beverage has been soothing folks for thousands of years, dating back to the ancient Romans, Egyptians, and Greeks. The world's first great healers—Hippocrates, Asclepius, Dioscorides, and Galen—all documented its use.

Back in the day, chamomile tea provided a medicine chest's worth of useful remedies. Its list of treatable conditions included cold-related symptoms, stomach and gastrointestinal problems, toothaches, convulsions, and insomnia. People used chamomile as a gargle or antiseptic wash and inhaled the tea's steam to reduce congestion and clear up irritations throughout the respiratory tract.

Historically, midwives treated pregnancy and childbirth issues with chamomile tea. Today, despite reservations that chamomile's effect on uterine muscles could stimulate uterine contractions, the tea is generally considered safe for

USE FOR

Acne

Anal itching

Arthritis

Belching

Blisters

Body odor

Colic

Diarrhea

Digestive problems

Gum problems

Headache

Healthy skin

Hives

Insomnia

Menstrual cramps

Morning sickness

Nausea

Shingles

Sore throat

Stings and bites

Ulcers

pregnant women. Healers also soaked poultices in a hot chamomile infusion to soothe back pain, gout, earaches, skin inflammations, bruises, and arthritis.

what's in it?

Chamomile contains a handful of major healing components. Among them are chamazulene and alpha-bisabolol. Chamazulene, formed during the heating of the tea or extract, has proven anti-inflammatory activity. Alpha-bisabolol is antibacterial, antifungal, and anti-inflammatory, and can promote the healing of ulcers, burns, and eczema. Chamomile's volatile oils help expel digestive gas, relax muscles, kill bacteria, and have a sedative effect.

what science says

Recently, science proved that the ancients were right on target when they prescribed chamomile tea to calm frayed nerves. In 2009, researchers from the University of Pennsylvania conducted a gold standard clinical trial (meaning that it was placebo-controlled and neither the researchers nor the participants knew whether they were getting a real or a sham treatment) to study chamomile's effects on people with generalized anxiety disorder. Fifty-seven people with mild to moderate anxiety disorder took either chamomile as an extract or a fake treatment daily for eight weeks. The researchers reported that folks in the chamomile group had significantly improved scores—meaning

A soothing bedtime story

Chamomile tea's ability to calm jangled nerves was immortalized in Beatrix Potter's famous children's story *The Tale of Peter Rabbit,* treasured by children for more than 100 years. Against his mother's wishes, little Peter sneaks into Mr. McGregor's garden, eats too much, is chased by McGregor, and catches a chill while hiding in a watering can. When Peter arrives home, he doesn't feel well. His mother puts him to bed early with a dose of chamomile tea—"one tablespoonful to be taken at bedtime"—which is still a common remedy for ailing and anxious children.

they were less anxious—on standardized tests than those who took the sham treatment.

enjoy a cup (or three) of comfort

When you drink chamomile tea regularly (two or three cups every day), it can protect against peptic ulcers; ease irritable bowel syndrome, indigestion, and stomach cramps; and act as a gentle, natural tranquilizer. What's more, chamomile tea can prevent muscle spasms and relax the smooth muscles that line the internal organs, such as the stomach and the uterus, making it a good remedy for easing stomach upsets and menstrual cramps.

Even though chamomile flowers contain pollen and may cause an allergic reaction when ingested or applied externally, researchers have found that chamomile may have antiallergenic properties. The potential effect is attributed to the as-yet-unconfirmed histamine-blocking action of chemical compounds called azulenes.

cinnamon

Cinnamon (*Cinnamomum verum*) comes from the bark of a small tree native to Asia, and it's been revered for its healing power for nearly 5,000 years, making it one of the world's oldest natural remedies. Chefs around the world rely on cinnamon for the distinctive flavor that enhances dishes, both sweet and savory. Today, cinnamon has captured the attention of researchers who've learned that it can be a powerful tool for helping balance blood sugar.

rooted in history

The first healer to write about cinnamon back in 2800 BC or so was Shen Nung, known as the father of Chinese medicine. In Egypt, cinnamon was among the several spices used for mummification. The Phoenicians and Hebrews called it "qinamon," and it was mentioned in the Hebrew Bible in Exodus (chapter 30, verse 23).

By the time the Europeans discovered cinnamon around the first century, it was so prized that 350 grams of the stuff cost 15 times more than silver. In the Middle Ages, cinnamon was used as a remedy for coughs and indigestion, though only by the wealthy—it was still wildly expensive. Historically, healers have recommended the spice for an amazing and diverse collection of human ills, including kidney trouble, bed-wetting, morning sickness, rheumatism, heart pain, warts, and toothaches.

what's in it?

Cinnamon is rich in essential oils that contain active medicinal compounds, including cinnamaldehyde, cinnamyl acetate, and cinnamyl alcohol. Collectively, these have significant antibacterial and antifungal action—so much so that research shows that cinnamon can be as effective as chemical food preservatives. Cinnamaldehyde prevents blood platelets from clumping, which means that cinnamon can help protect you against strokes and heart attacks. Cinnamon is also known as a powerful antioxidant that helps lessen inflammation.

what science says

Recently, scientists discovered that cinnamon lowers blood sugar levels in people who have type 2 diabetes and reduces heart disease risks for overweight people. In 2009, the American College of Nutrition published a study that helped clarify how cinnamon accomplishes this. In the study, conducted by a researcher from the U.S. Department of Agriculture, 22 overweight and obese people were given either 250 milligrams of cinnamon or a placebo twice a day for 12 weeks. The fasting blood sugar of those in the cinnamon group dropped from 114 to 102 mg/dL—a very healthy decline. The fasting blood sugar of the people in the placebo group increased a bit, from 112 to 113 mg/dL.

Many of cinnamon's traditional uses have been put to the test of science. Recent studies, for example, demonstrate its ability to stimulate the gastrointestinal tract, lending support to folk healers' long-held belief that the spice eases gas, nausea, vomiting, and other forms of gastrointestinal distress. That cinnamon is also a powerful antiseptic is no longer simply a matter of folk wisdom. A Japanese study demonstrated its ability to kill fungi, bacteria, and other microorganisms, including the bacteria that cause botulism and staph infections.

cranberry juice

Don't exile cranberries to the holiday relish plate—enjoy them year-round as juice, a dried snack fruit, and a tasty toss-in for cereals, muffins, and other baked goods. Cranberries belong to the same family as blueberries, and like them, are packed to the brim with antioxidants. As a home remedy, you can rely on cranberry juice to fight bladder infections.

USE FOR

Added antioxidants

Bladder infections

Cystitis prevention

Fatigue

Gout

Kidney and
  bladder stones

Urinary tract
  infections

rooted in history

If ever there was an all-American fruit, it's the cranberry. Native Americans cooked them and ate them sweetened with honey and maple syrup, a dish that certainly could have been served at the Pilgrim's first Thanksgiving dinner. Healers used them medicinally in poultices for wounds, and this probably was fairly effective. Cranberries are rich in tannins, which would have helped stop bleeding, and they contain compounds with antibiotic effects that would have prevented wounds from becoming infected.

what's in it?

Cranberries contain antioxidants, some of which come from proanthocyanidins (which give the berries their vivid color). These neutralize the particles in the body called free radicals. Like tiny Pac-Man characters, free radicals careen through the body and damage cell membranes and DNA—and can even cause cell death. Eating a variety of brightly colored fruits and vegetables ensures that you get a broad spectrum of antioxidants, which cuts your risks for developing a host of chronic diseases, including cancer, heart disease, and diabetes.

what science says

Studies have shown that drinking cranberry juice regularly can decrease the number of urinary tract infections in women who are prone to them, by inhibiting the ability of the *E. coli* bacteria to adhere to bladder walls. Interestingly, a study conducted at Harvard Medical School showed that eating a 1.5-ounce serving of sweetened dried cranberries might also be able to inhibit bacterial adherence and could potentially also help prevent UTIs.

top remedy for bladder problems

Cranberry juice has long been used as a home remedy for cystitis and to prevent kidney and bladder stones. Originally, this benefit was attributed to quinic acid, a cranberry substance that increases urine acidity and prevents the formation of calcium stones. Researchers thought that this acidity helped prevent cystitis. Studies show, however, that cranberries also contain a natural antibiotic substance that makes the bladder walls inhospitable to the organisms responsible for urinary tract infections. This prevents the bacteria from forming colonies; instead, they are washed out of the body in the urine. (Blueberry juice has a similar protective effect.)

BUYER'S tip

Most commercial cranberry juice is too diluted to be effective in preventing or treating urinary tract infections. It also contains large amounts of sugar or other sweeteners. Use a juicer to make your own cranberry juice. To reduce the amount of sugar needed, dilute a cup of freshly squeezed juice with 2 to 3 cups of apple juice, then sweeten to taste if necessary. You can buy organic, unsweetened cranberry juice in health food stores. Mix a little with club soda for a tart, refreshing drink.

Good to Know

Alas, the majority of cranberry juice products on a grocery store shelf are actually "cocktail" blends that contain precious few cranberries and more sweeteners than in soda. To get the health benefits of cranberries, get 100-percent pure cranberry juice.

flaxseed

Flaxseed (*Linum usitatissimum*) has been called a super-food—and with good reason. It's amazing how powerfully healthy these tiny seeds are. Harvested from the same plant that has supplied the fiber for linen since the dawn of time, flaxseed should be thought of as your strong-armed ally against high cholesterol, heart disease, symptoms of menopause, and even some forms of cancer. Make sure it has a permanent place in your pantry.

rooted in history

Flax is one of the world's oldest cultivated plants; people have grown it for its fiber, oil, and seeds for something like 10,000 years. The first record of its food use dates back to 3000 BC in Babylonia. Its medicinal use was first recorded, so far as we know, by Hippocrates, the father of medicine, who used flax to relieve intestinal discomfort. Roman healers relied on flax to ease coughs, urinary tract problems, and constipation.

North American healers, back in the day, used crushed flaxseed as a poultice for abscesses, ulcers, and inflammations. Linseed oil, a flaxseed product, was a popular cough syrup ingredient. And flaxseed tea, with a little lemon and honey, was often recommended for coughs and colds.

what's in it?

Flaxseed is a bountiful source of phytoestrogens called lignans, which act like a weak form of estrogen in the body. Lignans block estrogen receptors on cells—which means they prevent the uptake of stronger, pro-cancer estrogen—and may contribute to reduced rates of certain hormone-related cancers, including ovarian, breast, and prostate cancer. Other anticancer benefits have been attributed to lignans' ability to lower tumor necrosis factor, a protein compound involved in the inflammatory process.

And that's not all. Flax is an abundant source of alpha-linolenic acid (ALA), an essential fatty acid the body uses to make omega-3 fatty acids. ALA thins the blood and makes it less sticky, thus reducing the risk of heart attack and stroke. The little seeds also lower cholesterol, thanks to their big stores of soluble fiber: A tablespoon of ground flaxseed sprinkled over cereal or yogurt provides an easy 2.3 grams of fiber. Flaxseed's anti-inflammatory power may also help keep various conditions, from acne to asthma, at bay.

what science says

According to a 2009 study published in the *American Journal of Clinical Nutrition*, postmenopausal women and people who have high cholesterol could lower their cholesterol significantly simply by adding flaxseed to their diets. The researchers reviewed 28 studies on flax published between 1990 and 2008 before arriving at their conclusion.

on the horizon

When researchers study flaxseed and its potential for reducing the incidence of cancer, intriguing—and hopeful—evidence often emerges. For example, studies suggest that flaxseed and other foods rich in lignans (which include barley, oatmeal, and wheat bran) are potent cancer fighters. A flax-supplemented diet prevented breast cancer and slowed the growth and spread of malignant tumors in animal studies.

What's more, animal research shows that flaxseed also appears to increase the effectiveness of tamoxifen, a drug that reduces the risk of breast cancer by interfering with estrogen. Some studies suggest that flaxseed may prevent other forms of cancer that are fed by hormones, including prostate cancer.

While the research is exciting, little of it involves humans. A few studies have found that women who consume the most lignans have a lower-than-expected risk of

BUYER's tip

To add flaxseed to your diet, buy it in bulk at a natural foods store, and keep it in an airtight container in the pantry. Pick up a coffee grinder and grind the amount you need every day, because ground flaxseed is highly perishable. If you grind too much, refrigerate the excess in a plastic bag and use promptly.

Researchers see hopeful evidence that flaxseed can help reduce the incidence of cancer.

breast cancer, though the benefit may be limited to women who have not reached menopause. Until more studies are completed, it's too soon to call flaxseed a cancer fighter. However, its other benefits make it a smart food to eat regularly, so if flax does turn out to fight cancer, you can consider it a bonus.

flaxseed oil

Just as olives are different than olive oil, so is flaxseed different than flaxseed oil. In particular, flaxseed oil doesn't contain the lignans that appear so useful on the cancer front. However, flaxseed oil is 50 to 60 percent alpha-linolenic acid (ALA), an essential omega-3 fatty acid. Unlike other well-known omega-3 oils—like eicosapentaenoic acid (EPA) and docosahexaenoic acid (DHA), which are found in fish—ALA comes strictly from plants.

Buy flaxseed oil at health-food stores. The best products are made with fresh-pressed seeds, bottled in opaque containers, and processed at low temperatures. The oil is highly perishable and needs to be refrigerated. Don't cook with flaxseed oil; use it raw as a salad dressing or veggie drizzle or an ingredient in smoothies and other recipes that don't require heating.

Good to Know

If you're a woman past menopause or have diabetes, read on. News about flaxseed oil that emerged in 2009 offers hope about avoiding osteoporosis. Researchers at the National Research Center in Cairo, Egypt, studied the effect of diabetes on bone health to see whether flaxseed oil could delay the onset of the bone-weakening disease. One key finding: that diabetes puts post-menopausal women at increased risk for osteoporosis. The researchers concluded that flaxseed oil improves bone health and could prevent osteoporosis. The study was conducted on lab rats, so human studies need to confirm this effect in women. Bottom line: Since flaxseed oil's other health benefits are well-proven, it certainly makes sense to add a spoonful or two to veggies and salads in hopes of preventing osteoporosis, especially if you're at risk for the disease.

garlic

More health benefits have been ascribed to garlic (*Allium sativum*) than to just about any other food—and with good reason. The short list of reasons why it's smart to be a frequent garlic eater include its antibiotic action, its ability to foil respiratory ailments in the making, and its potential for boosting the health of your heart and protecting you against certain cancers.

rooted in history

Could garlic be the secret that helped raise the great pyramids? It's possible: The Egyptians rationed it to pyramid builders to boost their strength (and to help prevent dysentery). Meanwhile, across the Red Sea, a garlic prescription written in cuneiform was discovered on a Sumerian clay tablet dating back to 3000 BC. Chinese and Indian healers wrote of using garlic as a blood thinner back in 1500 BC. Hippocrates reportedly used garlic to treat cervical cancer. In the early 1700s, French gravediggers drank a brew of crushed garlic and wine in hopes of warding off the plague.

Garlic's first investigator was none other than Louis Pasteur, the great French scientist. He discovered its antibacterial and antifungal powers in the mid-1800s. Later, at his hospital in Africa, Albert Schweitzer used garlic to treat dysentery.

Finally, garlic played a helpful patriotic role during World Wars I and II, when soldiers were given the stuff to prevent gangrene.

USE FOR

Athlete's foot
Cancer protection
Colds and flu
Earache
Gastrointestinal ailments
High blood pressure
High cholesterol
Improved immunity
Respiratory infections
Ringworm
Sinusitis
Swimmer's ear
Ulcers
Urinary tract infections
Warts
Yeast infections

BUYER'S tip

Good to Know

Eating five or more cloves a day can result in heartburn, flatulence, and intestinal distress. Because garlic is a blood thinner, people taking aspirin or anticoagulant drugs, as well as people with clotting disorders, should check with their doctors before taking medicinal amounts of garlic. In rare cases, garlic may cause an allergic reaction.

Since drying alters the active ingredients of fresh garlic, don't substitute dried powdered garlic when using garlic medicinally.

what's in it?

A garlic bulb is a virtual chemical factory full of substances that are highly volatile. Because they're so unstable, their health benefits depend on how fresh the garlic is, and whether it's been crushed, chopped, chewed, or cooked. Among these are sulfur compounds including thiosulfinates, which are responsible for garlic's distinctive aroma and for many of its effects. Garlic's heart-protective ability has recently been attributed to a chemical called S-allylcysteine.

Another active component is a substance called alliin. When a clove is crushed, bruised, or chewed, the alliin is converted into allicin, which cannot survive the heat of cooking or the acid in your stomach. But when you chew fresh garlic, the allicin (and its benefits) is quickly absorbed in your mouth.

Garlic has antibacterial, antimicrobial, and antifungal activity, which in addition to its other benefits, makes it a great home remedy for healing wounds and athlete's foot and for expelling worms.

what science says

Garlic studies published in 2008 and 2009 confirm that garlic lowers cholesterol and blood pressure and helps prevent the common cold, and that a diet rich in the pungent stuff can reduce the risk for prostate and other cancers.

Also recently, researchers from the University of Connecticut ended confusion about the best way to use garlic. They discovered that freshly crushed garlic, rather than garlic that's been processed or cooked, is best for helping protect against heart attacks.

the heart-protecting bulb

When eaten daily, garlic can help lower heart disease risk by as much as 76 percent. It performs this miraculous feat by moderately reducing cholesterol levels (by between 5 and 10 percent in some studies), by thinning the blood and thereby staving off dangerous clots, and by acting as an antioxidant. Garlic's sulfur compounds also appear to ward off cancer, especially stomach and colorectal cancer. The compounds flush out carcinogens before they can damage cell DNA, and they force cancer cells that do develop to self-destruct.

ginger

Inexpensive, fast acting, scientifically proven, and delicious are terrific attributes for a home remedy to have. And when it comes to easing motion sickness and nausea, ginger is all of those—and more. Ginger (*Zingiber officinale*) has a track record for attacking inflammation and easing pain, both excellent reasons to make sure this rhizome has a dedicated space in your kitchen medicine cabinet.

rooted in history

People have been spicing up their foods with ginger for over 4,000 years. One of its first fans, in fact, was Confucius, who legendarily added it to everything he ate. Ancient Chinese, Indian, Roman, and Grecian healers wrote about the gnarly root's medicinal value, and the list of ills they pitted it against is a long one. Once early North American medics discovered ginger, they used it in warm baths to soothe bruises and tired muscles. As a home remedy, folks chewed gingerroot to soothe sore throats and grated it into olive oil as an antidandruff potion. Warm ginger compresses were an old-time treatment for soothing sinus congestion, menstrual cramps, and general aches and fatigue.

what's in it?

Researchers have identified more than 400 chemicals in gingerroot, though we know about the medicinal properties of only a handful of them. Ginger's antinausea and anti-vomiting properties are likely due to the compounds

USE FOR

Arthritis

Back pain

Belching

Bursitis and
tendinitis

Colds and flu

Coughs

Dandruff

Fever

Flatulence

Hangover

Indigestion

Migraines

Menstrual cramps

Morning sickness

Motion sickness

Nausea and
vomiting

Sinusitis

Stomachaches

Toothache

Ulcers

6-gingerol, 6-shogaol, and galanolactone. Scientists believe that they may act on the brain's "vomiting center" to subdue the urge to vomit. They also work in the digestive tract to ease the sensation of nausea.

Gingerols, shogaols, and another compound, paradols, are behind ginger's anti-inflammatory actions. The powerful antioxidant 6-gingerol inhibits production of nitric oxide, which forms a really nasty free radical called peroxynitrite that's known to cause cell death. Inhibiting this free radical is proven to ease inflammation and pain and to improve diseases that affect blood vessels. In fact, gingerols act like the COX-II selective, nonsteroidal anti-inflammatory drugs (NSAIDs) such as Celebrex, which explains why ginger has been clinically proven to ease osteoarthritis pain. Unlike NSAIDs, however, ginger has no toxic side effects.

what science says

Recently, scientists have learned more about ginger's ability to suppress cancer cells, an action researchers have been studying for years. In one 2009 study, researchers from the University of Minnesota discovered that 6-gingerol, one of the herb's active compounds, suppressed the growth of colorectal tumors in lab mice. And on a test of human breast cancer cells conducted in the lab, researchers in Korea demonstrated that 6-gingerol inhibited the cells' ability to metastasize, or spread, to other parts of the body.

Iranian researchers recently studied ginger's ability to lower cholesterol. When they gave ginger or a placebo to people with high cholesterol for 45 days, those who took the ginger had lower levels of LDL (unhealthy) cholesterol and higher levels of HDL (healthy) cholesterol than did the people who took the placebo.

Research has also proven that ginger reduces pain and swelling in people with arthritis. It may work against migraines by blocking inflammatory substances called prostaglandins.

And then there are the digestive benefits. In the early 1980s, American scientists began reporting that ginger prevents motion sickness better than popular commercial products. Subsequent research in the United States, Sweden, Germany, and Britain confirms that ginger reduces dizziness, anesthesia-related nausea, and the vomiting and cold sweats associated with seasickness.

honey

Honey is truly one of nature's sweetest miracles. Tiny bees, zipping along at up to 15 miles an hour, zoom as far as nine miles away to search for nectar. During just one nectar foray, bees may visit 100 flowers. Sweeter than sugar, honey's thick, syrupy texture makes it the perfect home remedy for easing coughs and sore throats, while its high sugar content makes it a natural antibiotic.

rooted in history

Honey just might be the world's oldest home remedy; bees have been producing the stuff for at least 100 million years. Written references to honey date back 7,500 years or so to Egypt and Sumeria. Of the 900 known remedies in ancient Egyptian medicine, 500 contained honey. In the first century, Pliny the Elder recorded his cure for dropsy and bladder stones in a recipe that included honey and powdered bees. It's been written that ancient Olympians dined on honey and figs to enhance their athletic performance.

By medieval times, honey's medicinal use was mostly limited to its ability to make medicines taste a little less terrible, and it was also used externally to heal wounds. Hundreds of years later, honey found its way into recipes for patent medicines all over the world.

what science says

Science has focused its attention on honey's wound-healing ability. A small study conducted in the United Kingdom

USE FOR

Acne
Allergies
Anxiety
Chapped lips
Colds and flu
Conjunctivitis
Constipation
Coughs
Cuts and scrapes
Eczema
Hangovers
Healthy skin
Heartburn
Hiccups
Indigestion
Laryngitis
Psoriasis
Shingles
Ulcers

showed that Manuka honey (a New Zealand variety) healed wounds from radiation therapy that had not responded to conventional treatments. In another recent study conducted in the United Kingdom, the wounds of 105 patients were treated either with honey or a conventional dressing. After 12 weeks, the honey treatment healed wounds 12 percent faster than did the conventional dressing.

Turns out that honey is more than a sweet addition to cough syrups. In one study, conducted by researchers at Pennsylvania State University, honey improved coughs better than dextromethorphan (DM), a common ingredient in many cough suppressants.

what's in it?

You won't be surprised to learn that honey is mostly made up of sugars—38.2 percent fructose, 31 percent glucose; disaccharides such as sucrose and maltose and oligosaccharides made up the rest. That honey is laced with beneficial substances is clear: In a new study, some of the phytonutrients found in raw honey were shown to prevent colon cancer in lab animals.

Honey also contains antioxidants, including one called pinocembrin. Chinese test-tube and animal studies showed that pinocembrin seems to protect brain cells. Whether it has a similar effect in humans is as yet unknown. Other honey antioxidants include quercetin, kaempferol, and apigenin.

gentle wound healer

Honey's high sugar content, combined with its hydrogen peroxide and propolis (a compound in nectar that kills bacteria) content, pulls moisture from wounds, denies bacteria the moisture they need to survive, and locks out harmful external contaminants—actions that help wounds heal faster.

In the days before antibiotics, infection was the greatest health threat. Even small wounds could turn deadly, which is why doctors often carried honey in their black bags. Even now that triple-antibiotic creams are in every medicine chest, some doctors believe that honey might be a superior wound dressing in some cases. It works so well that a number of manufacturers sell honey-impregnated dressings for hard-to-heal wounds.

lemon

You get more than a tart blast when you suck on a slice of lemon or sip lemonade. Lemons are an extraordinarily rich source of healing compounds that improve immunity, strengthen blood vessels, and help skin heal. They may even block cell changes that can lead to cancer. A generous squeeze or two of lemon and a spoonful of honey in a cup of hot water is the perfect sore throat elixir. Lemon is also an indispensable ingredient for concocting homemade cough syrups and DIY beauty treatments.

rooted in history

Originally developed as a cross between a fruit called the citron and the lime, lemons probably originated in China or India some 2,500 years ago. Arabs introduced them to Spain and North Africa around the 11th century, and the Crusaders helped spread them through the rest of Europe. Christopher Columbus brought them to the Americas on his second voyage in 1493, and they've been grown in Florida since the 1500s. Centuries ago, British sailors ate lemons by the boatload to prevent scurvy, a deadly disease caused by vitamin C deficiency. A single lemon packs 39 milligrams of vitamin C, more than half the Recommended Dietary Allowance.

Miners and pioneers also relied on lemons to fight scurvy during the California gold rush, and valued them so highly that they'd pay as much as one dollar a lemon back in 1849, a huge sum back then for a tiny fruit—in today's money, that's about $25.58.

USE FOR

Acne

Allergies

Age spots

Antiseptic

Body odor

Calluses and corns

Colds and flu

Constipation

Coughs

Energy

Fever

Indigestion

Healthy skin

Heartburn

Kidney stones

Mood enhancement

Morning sickness

Motion sickness

Sinusitis

Sore throat

Varicose veins

what's in it?

The vitamin C in lemons lowers levels of histamine, the chemical that contributes to stuffy noses and runny eyes. The vitamin is a powerful antioxidant that also reduces levels of free radicals, those nasty cell-damaging molecules, and helps guard against heart disease. (Several studies have shown that low levels of vitamin C increase the risk for heart attacks. When cholesterol becomes oxidized—attacked by free radicals—it's more likely to turn into artery-clogging plaque.) The body uses vitamin C to boost the activity of immune cells and manufacture collagen, the tissue-building substance that assists in wound healing.

Lemons are also loaded with citric acid, a chemical that reduces calcium excretion and helps prevent the forma-tion of kidney stones. If kidney stones are an issue for you, consider drinking eight 8-ounce glasses of lemonade made with fresh lemon juice daily (sweetened with as little sugar as possible). This refreshing drink prevents the formation of kidney stones as effectively as do prescription citrate drugs, such as potassium citrate.

Finally, lemon zest is rich in a bioflavonoid (a group of antioxidant plant chemicals) called rutin, which strength-ens the walls of the veins and capillaries and reduces the pain—and even the occurrence—of varicose veins.

BUYER's tip

Look for unblemished lemons with a rich yellow color and smooth skin. Coarse or rough texture often indicates the skin is thick, meaning less flesh and juice inside. Another buyer's trick is sensing the weight: the heavier it feels, the better. Before you juice them, roll them on a flat surface with the palm of your hand. This helps them yield more juice.

mustard

The tiny seeds of this leafy broccoli and cabbage relative make one of the most popular condiments of all time. But mustard is much more than a taste bud perker-upper. Healers have known for ages that mustard's pungent heat thins mucus and makes it easier to breathe when you have a cold or flu. What's more, mustard contains a variety of chemical compounds with impressive healing credentials.

rooted in history

To the ancients, mustard was practically a panacea. Egyptian, Sumerian, and Chinese healers all used mustard seeds as medicine. The famous Greek physician Dioscorides counted on mustard to treat conditions as diverse as epilepsy and tonsillitis, and the early Romans chewed the seeds to ease toothache pain and used mustard ointments to treat stings. But the most famous mustard remedy is the mustard plaster, which dates back to Hippocrates, the father of medicine, as a treatment for lung problems and rheumatism. It's a testament to its success that healers in countries all over the world have relied on mustard plasters for a long list of ailments. However, we cringe at one of its uses: In 18th-century Russia, mustard plasters were administered as a treatment for mental illness.

what's in it?

Mustard seeds are loaded with phytonutrients called glucosinolates, which are responsible for mustard's spiciness. They help protect against colon and rectal cancer. What's

USE FOR

Athlete's foot

Arthritis pain

Back pain

Belching

Bursitis and tendinitis

Chest congestion

Colds and flu

Fever

Headache

Ringworm

more, mustard seeds rank as good sources of omega-3 fatty acids, tryptophan, selenium, and magnesium—but you'd have to eat a two-teaspoon sized serving of mustard seeds to reap those nutritional benefits. Finally, mustard seeds contain hefty doses of myrosin and sinigrin, chemicals that make mucus watery and easier to expel from the body.

the warming remedy

Herbalists call mustard a rubefacient, meaning that it stimulates circulation, which creates soothing warmth when you apply it to the skin. Like cayenne pepper, it also appears to deplete nerve cells of substance P, a chemical that transmits pain signals back to the brain. Soaking your feet in hot water with a little mustard powder is the ultimate multitasking remedy: It can unblock a stuffed head, help ease fever, and soothe a headache—all by drawing blood to the feet. This eases the pressure on the blood vessels in your head, helps disperse congestion, and increases circulation.

A traditional congestion remedy is to apply a mustard plaster—made by crushing a few tablespoonfuls of mustard seeds and adding them to a cup of flour or cornmeal along with a little water to make a paste—to your chest. The aroma unclogs nasal stuffiness, while the "heat" increases blood circulation in the chest and makes it easier to breathe. Just don't leave the plaster on too long (usually no more than 15 minutes) or it will burn the skin. You can protect the skin before you put the plaster on by applying a coating of petroleum jelly. Be sure to wash your hands thoroughly after handling a mustard plaster and before touching your eyes, nose, or mouth.

BUYER'S tip

Three kinds of mustard seeds are available: those from the black (*Brassica nigra*), white (*Brassica alba*) and brown (*Brassica juncea*) mustard plants. Black mustard seeds have the sharpest flavor. White mustard seeds are actually yellow and are used to make American mustard and yellow mustard powder. Brown seeds are used to make Dijon and other brown mustards. For the remedies in this book, buy white (yellow) mustard seeds and grind them in a coffee grinder or buy mustard power, such as Coleman's.

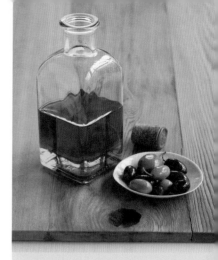

olive oil

Nutritionists have sung the praises of the Mediterranean diet for so long that it's easy to forget how radical the idea was that certain fats, like olive oil, could actually be good for your heart. But the evidence was strong: In the mid-1980s, a long-term study comparing rates of cardiovascular disease in seven countries revealed that heart attacks were relatively uncommon in countries where the people consumed lots of olive oil, including Italy and Greece. Since then, scores of clinical studies have left little doubt that olive oil protects the cardiovascular system.

rooted in history

Olives grow where little else survives—hot, dry climates suit olive trees just fine. So it's no surprise that the first olive oil probably came from a Mediterranean country like Syria, Lebanon, Palestine, or Israel. The ancients put a high price on their olive oil—in ancient Syria, around 2000 BC, its value was five times that of wine. But that probably had to do with its use as a lamp oil.

Olive oil figured prominently into religious rites and rituals. It was used to consecrate the dead and to anoint royalty and warriors. In fact, the word Messiah means "the anointed one." The ancients used olive oil for medicinal ointments, in beauty concoctions, to give skin and hair a healthy glow, and to make soap. In the world's first cookbook, *De Re Coquinaria* (Cooking Matters), by the Roman gourmet Apicius, olive oil is among the 10 most common ingredients in the book's 468 recipes.

USE FOR

Allergies

Asthma

Back pain

Brittle nails

Cancer risk reduction

Chapped lips

Clear skin

Eczema

Head lice

Heart health

High blood pressure

High cholesterol

Infection prevention

Menstrual symptoms

Moisturizer

Nosebleed

Psoriasis

Sore feet

what science says

Scientists have known for decades that people whose diets are rich in olive oil have low rates of heart disease. Now they've figured out more about how the golden green liquid works its magic.

Scientists have long known that a diet rich in olive oil protects the heart. Now they are finally discovering how.

In a recent study, Spanish researchers reported that when people ate olive oil-enriched Mediterranean-style diets for a year, their blood pressure dropped significantly. People in the study whose Mediterranean-style diets were enriched with nuts also dropped a bit, but people in a third group, on a basic low-fat diet, experienced no blood pressure changes. People in the olive oil group also experienced a substantial drop in their levels of C-reactive protein (an inflammation marker linked to heart disease) compared to people in the other two groups. (The C-reactive protein levels of those in the low-fat group actually rose.) The most fascinating thing to come out of this study? Olive oil seems to change the structure of red blood cells, which the researchers speculated could account for its ability to lower cholesterol and blood pressure.

Also recently, Italian researchers compared over 20,000 cases of people with cancer to 18,000 healthy people. They discovered that people whose diets included olive oil and other healthy fats had a lower cancer risk.

Finally, Spanish researchers in 2009 followed men with severely high cholesterol, all of whom were taking the cholesterol-lowering drug simvastatin, for six months. There were two groups: men whose diets contained olive oil or men who used sunflower oil. Men in the olive oil

Good to Know

Yes, olives are great for you, too, and make a fine snack in moderation. Most olives are inedible straight from the tree; they need to be cured to remove certain bitter chemicals. The variations between olives all relate to their ripeness at harvest, the curing process used, and their exposure to air during the curing process (air is one way to turn an olive dark). The only health caveat for olives is saltiness: Some types are overloaded with the stuff. If you love olives but can't handle the salt, give them a rinse before eating.

group lowered their total cholesterol more than did the men in the sunflower oil group, leading the researchers to advise that people with high cholesterol use olive oil instead of sunflower oil, even if they're taking effective cholesterol-lowering medications.

oil that acts like heart medicine

Still other studies show that olive oil acts a bit like aspirin, reducing levels of chronic low-grade inflammation, another culprit behind heart attacks. Finally, olive oil is teeming with antioxidants, which act on cholesterol to make it less likely to stick to artery walls. Olive oil is rich in unique disease-fighting phytochemicals, vitamin E, and mono-unsaturated fat, which all help to clear cholesterol from arteries. The antioxidant phytochemicals hydroxytyrosol and oleuropein may work together, according to laboratory studies, to help protect against breast cancer, high blood pressure, infection-causing bacteria, and heart disease. Lignans, present in extra-virgin olive oil, may protect against cancer by suppressing early cancer changes in cells.

the best press

The heat and chemicals used in processing olive oil can diminish its nutrient content, which is why it's best to choose minimally processed oils, such as extra-virgin, cold-pressed oil.

Virgin olive oil is the oily juice pressed from the olive. It is unrefined. The term virgin refers to oils that are slightly more acidic than the extra-virgin ones; they must contain no more than 3 grams of free oleic acid per 100 grams.

Extra-virgin olive oil is the least acidic and has a maximum acid level of 1 gram of free oleic acid per 100 grams of oil. It's the choice of chefs because it offers the widest variety of flavors and aromas and has a "fruity" flavor.

The flavor differences are due to the regions where the olives are cultivated, the climate, the variety of olive, and to some degree the manner in which the olives are harvested. Steer clear of bottles labeled "extra light" and "light." These olive oils are the most refined, yet are no lower in calories or fat. They lack the flavor and many of the benefits of the extra-virgin olive oils.

peppermint

Count on sprightly peppermint (*Mentha piperita*) as your go-to herb for easing upset stomachs and minor digestive woes. The oils it contains, especially menthol and menthone, relax the smooth muscles that line the intestinal tract, helping to relieve cramping. Menthol's decongestant, mucus-thinning action makes it a smart addition to remedies for colds and coughs. Mint is also a wonderful ingredient in home remedies for soothing itchy skin irritations.

rooted in history

As Greek myth has it, when the god Pluto fell in love with the nymph Menthe, his wife, Proserpine, fell into a fit of jealous rage and—poof! She changed Menthe into the plant we now call mint. Based on the myth's romance, the ancient Greek philosopher Theophrastus officially gave mint its botanical name, menthe.

Early Romans cooked with mint, and the Greeks used it as a restorative, much like smelling salts. England's great 17th-century herbalist Nicholas Culpeper called mint "singularly good" for some 40 different health problems. Among them, he recommended it for headaches, a use that one small 1994 study has confirmed.

what's in it?

More than 100 components have been identified in mint. As with all medicinal plants, their exact composition

USE FOR

Acne

Arthritis

Belching

Body odor

Colds and flu

Coughs

Extra energy

Fatigue

Flatulence

Foot problems

Headache

Indigestion

Irritable bowel
    syndrome

Morning sickness

Nausea and
    vomiting

Pain relief

Sinusitis

Skin care

Sore throat

Stings and bites

varies somewhat, depending on where and how the plant was grown and its particular variety—there are hundreds of mints. In general, mints contain the volatile oil menthol, which relaxes intestinal spasms, eases abdominal pain, and acts as a decongestant and topical pain reliever. It also contains the flavonoids rutin, luteolin, hesperidin, and eriocitrin, which have antiviral and antioxidant properties.

what science says

As a digestive aid, mint is hard to beat—even though relatively few clinical studies have been conducted on the herb. Instead of looking at the herb itself, most studies have focused on peppermint oil and its ability to ease symptoms of irritable bowel syndrome, or IBS.

Most recently, researchers at the Tehran University of Medical Sciences gave 90 people with IBS a placebo or a specially coated, delayed-release peppermint oil capsule three times a day for eight weeks. At the end of the study, 14 people who took the peppermint oil reported that they were free of pain or discomfort.

And in a Taiwanese study, IBS patients given peppermint-oil capsules 15 to 30 minutes before meals experienced significantly less bloating, stomach rumbling, and gas. Abdominal pain was reduced or eliminated entirely in some cases.

Good to Know

Peppermint is easy to grow—in fact, it's *too* easy. Experts recommend growing it in pots rather than in a bed because the plant often takes over a garden. Peppermint plants prefer full or partial sun and loamy soil. Use the leaves to make tea, flavor ice water, top ice cream, or add zest to vegetables and stir-fries.

BUYER'S tip

Find peppermint tea bags in supermarkets and health food stores; peppermint essential oil is sold in health food stores.

rosemary

If the only time you pull out your spice bottle of rosemary is when you're cooking lamb, you're missing out on a wonderful remedy for soothing nerves, boosting energy, and even enhancing memory. Rosemary (*Rosmarinus officinalis*) contains flavonoids with potent antioxidant action. These compounds may also strengthen blood vessels, can lessen inflammation, and may reduce the risk of cancers, arteriosclerosis, and other chronic diseases.

rooted in history

Rosemary's reputation as a memory-booster dates back to ancient Greece, when students would stick sprigs of it in their hair while studying for exams. And Grecian mourners would toss rosemary into graves as a symbol of remembrance. Thousands of years later, during the time of the Tudors, Sir Thomas More would write that he planted rosemary in his garden because it was "the herb sacred to remembrance." Even Shakespeare knew about rosemary's memory powers when he wrote these words for Hamlet's Ophelia: "There's rosemary, that's for remembrance."

Cosmetically, rosemary has been used to restore thinning hair. It was also a key ingredient in a concoction called "Queen of Hungary" water. History is a little murky about its actual creation, but for centuries, women used this rosemary-scented potion as a beauty lotion and perfume. An herbal book written in 1525 recommends rosemary boiled in wine as a facial wash.

USE FOR

Alertness

Anxiety

Arthritis

Body odor

Bruises

Cancer prevention

Concentration

Dandruff

Fatigue

Fever

Foot odor and pain

Hair loss

Headache

Memory

Muscle cramps

Varicose veins

what's in it?

Rosemary contains several flavonoids, including diosmin, diosmetin, genkwanin, and apigenin. Odd names aside, these white and yellow plant pigments have all been linked to beneficial actions in test tube studies. What we don't yet know, however, is how much rosemary you'd have to ingest to achieve those benefits. Still, the benefits are impressive. For example, apigenin can inhibit the growth of pancreatic cancer cells. Diosmin strengthens blood vessel walls. And genkwanin may help prevent wrinkles by triggering collagen production.

Other rosemary compounds include rosmarinic acid, which has anti-inflammatory and antioxidant properties. Rosemary extracts are also known to be antiviral.

Good to Know

Do not use rosemary medicinally if you are pregnant or breastfeeding.

what science says

In a recent study, researchers from Florida Atlantic University College of Nursing designed a method to test the effects of inhaling rosemary or lavender essential oil on anxiety and stress levels. They recruited 40 graduate nursing students and gave them an exam, and then measured their stress levels, pulse, and blood pressure. Then the volunteers took a second exam using a lavender inhaler, which they were instructed to sniff before and during the test. The students took a third test, using a rosemary inhaler.

The students said that when it came to test taking, rosemary was more helpful than lavender. It improved their recall and helped them stay alert during the test, the researchers reported. The lavender relaxed the students so well that it actually lessened their test-taking ability. The researchers concluded that rosemary heightens your awareness, improves concentration, and generally makes you more alert.

In a study conducted in 2007, Taiwanese scientists analyzed an extract of rosemary leaves and identified its five major compounds, which they then tested. Their findings led them to conclude that rosemary can be considered an "herbal anti-inflammatory and anti-tumor agent."

BUYER'S tip

Find dried rosemary leaves in the spice aisle of the supermarket. You can also buy it fresh in many markets, and it's a wonderful herb to grow in your garden.

sage

The herb you lace your Thanksgiving turkey stuffing with was prized for its medicinal power long before the Pilgrims landed at Plymouth Rock. Sage (*Salvia officinalis*) takes its scientific name from the Latin word *salvere*, which means "to be saved." That name is apt indeed: In pre-refrigeration days, sage was used to preserve meat. Healers consider it a handy remedy for digestive upsets, sore throats, colds, and sinusitis. And women transitioning through menopause often bless sage for its ability to reduce the dreaded night sweats.

rooted in history

Sage was sacred to the Romans, so much so that they even created a special ceremony for gathering it. In 1597, Gerard, the great British herbalist, wrote that sage was "singularly" good for the head and brain, quickened senses and memory, strengthened the sinews, and healed shaking and trembling. At least two old proverbs celebrate sage's medicinal value: "Why should a man die whilst sage grows in his garden," and, "He that would live for aye (forever) must eat sage in May."

what's in it?

Sage contains a complex blend of compounds, including diterpenes, which help give the herb its flavor and its health benefits. Of these, carnosic acid and carnosol (also found in rosemary) are antioxidants with anti-inflammatory properties. In lab studies, these two compounds appear to

USE FOR

Anxiety

Body odor

Canker sores

Colds and congestion

Concentration

Digestive problems

Foot problems

Healthy skin

High cholesterol

Laryngitis

Memory

Night sweats

Perspiration

Ringworm

Sinusitis

Sore throat

be able to lower blood sugar, though studies on humans are needed to confirm this action. Camphor is an anti-oxidant that kills fungi and bacteria, which explains sage's old use as a meat preservative. Other sage compounds are known to kill viruses.

what science says

In 2009, Portuguese researchers published a pilot study to see whether sage could lower blood glucose or cholesterol levels in healthy women. They gave six women 10 ounces of sage tea twice a day for four weeks. Though there were no effects on glucose levels, after eight weeks, the tea lowered the women's LDL (unhealthy) cholesterol by 12.4 percent, and increased their levels of HDL (healthy) cholesterol by 50.6 percent. What's more, drinking sage tea also raised blood levels of antioxidants. The researchers said that their study proves that sage tea is a safe and healthful beverage.

Sage reduces excess secretions from the sinuses and upper respiratory tract and also has a drying effect on excessive sweating—especially night sweats associated with menopause. Though there's only one study that supports this phenomenon, traditional herbalists frequently recommend sage for excess perspiration and night sweats.

Sage also improves memory, concentration, and anxiety. The results of a recent clinical trial, conducted on older adults, suggest that sage enhances attention as well as memory. In a 2006 study on healthy young adults, sage reduced anxiety and improved their performance when they took a test requiring them to "multitask."

Good to Know

Don't use sage medicinally when you're pregnant or breastfeeding, and don't give medicinal amounts to children.

BUYER's tip

Find dried sage in the spice aisle of your supermarket. Give it a sniff to make sure it's aromatic before you use it—that indicates freshness and potency. You can also find it fresh in many markets or easily grow it in your garden.

salt

You could say that as humans, all of us are "the salt of the earth"—not only the extra-good folks. That's because humans require from 5 to 10 grams of salt every day. Over a lifetime, a person might take in as much as 644 pounds of the stuff. Our bodies use salt, or sodium chloride, as an electrolyte, which is an electrically charged solution. This regulates the functioning of muscles and nerves and maintains our blood pressure, among many other critical operations.

rooted in history

Salt began to influence humans before the dawn of time. Neolithic settlements were founded at salt springs, and ever since our earliest days, salt has been an essential part of culture. In fact, controlling salt gave rise to three of the world's greatest civilizations: China, Egypt, and the Roman Empire. The Romans built one of their major roads, Via Salaria, or "salt road," from Rome to the Adriatic Sea to make it easier to transport the stuff. Roman soldiers were often paid in salt, and that's where the word "salary" comes from.

The earliest known book about drugs, published nearly 5,000 years ago in China, described over 40 kinds of salt, along with two methods for extracting and converting it—methods that are stunningly similar to modern-day techniques.

Since ancient times, salt helped people preserve and transport foods. Not only did salted foods keep longer, but salt dehydrated fish and meats and made them easier to ship. Finally, salt has played a key role in historic events, from the French Revolution to the Indian drive for independence from British rule.

the healing power of salt

It's no surprise that a substance linked so closely to life, both biologically and culturally, should have so many uses as a home remedy. Take simple salt water, for example. Because higher concentrations of sodium chloride draw water from surrounding tissues by osmosis, salt water helps soothe swollen gums and heal abscesses. Today, your dentist will tell you to rinse with warm salt water to ease gum irritation and speed healing. For generations, people suffering from head colds have relied on warm, diluted salt water, sniffed gently up the nostrils, to clear mucus from the nasal passages. And a salt-water gargle is a classic sore throat remedy.

Two teaspoons of salt in a pint of lukewarm water make a footbath that helps curb fungal infections by softening and cleansing the skin. Similarly, a salt-water soak makes it easier to remove a stubborn splinter. Salt water heated to body temperature may relieve earaches by loosening wax.

BUYER'S tip

When it comes to using salt in remedies, there's no difference between kosher salt, sea salt, or table salt. However, table salt will dissolve quicker.

tea

Think of those tea bags stashed in your kitchen cabinet as the ultimate life-extending home remedy. In particular, green tea has so many scientifically proven benefits that we wonder why everyone isn't drinking several cups a day. Though the word "tea" refers to all brews made with hot water and herbs, true tea is made from the leaves of an evergreen shrub, *Camellia sinensis*. Differences in the way the leaves are processed account for black, green, white, and oolong varieties. People who drink green tea lower their risk of dying from heart disease or stroke and have lower rates of heart disease, stroke, cancer, and even tooth decay. But don't neglect black or oolong teas. These hearty brews are also abundantly laced with disease-hindering antioxidants.

rooted in history

People have been brewing tea leaves for half a million years. The Chinese were among the first to cultivate the tea plant, which was considered medicinal as far back as 1046 BC. Chinese Taoists hailed tea as an "elixir of immortality," and artists and poets celebrated tea in their work. Utterly democratic in its appeal, tea was both an imperial tribute and a drink sold on street corners.

A Buddhist priest introduced the Japanese to a powdered green tea called matcha, which he'd discovered in China. Tea drinking then spread like wildfire throughout 12th-century Japan, and became essential to Japanese culture. It took Westerners hundreds of years to discover tea,

USE FOR

Acne

Anal itching

Arthritis

Boils

Cancer protection

Chicken pox

Cold sores

Colds and flu

Conjunctivitis

Coughs

Cuts

Diarrhea

Fatigue

Foot odor

Heart health

Hemorrhoids

Memory

Poison ivy/oak

Stings and bites

Stress

Sunburn

Toothache

Ulcers

but when they brought it back home from their first visits to Japan in the 1850s, it didn't create much interest, except in the Netherlands.

The Dutch eventually introduced tea to America, much to the delight of American colonists. Tea became such a hot colonial commodity that the British decided to tax and control it, a practice that inspired the historic act of defiance known as the Boston Tea Party.

what's in it?

Tea contains compounds called catechins. According to the National Cancer Institute, these profoundly healthy plant chemicals are potent antioxidants with antiviral and potential anti-cancer benefits. One tea catechin, known as EGCG, is 100 times more powerful than vitamin C—and it protects the DNA in cells from cancer-inducing changes. Although the highest concentration of catechins is found in green tea, black tea is also a good source. Brand-name teas are mixtures of as many as 20 different varieties of leaves, blended to ensure a consistent flavor.

what science says

The science doesn't get much clearer than this: Drinking black tea beats water when it comes to health benefits, say British nutrition researchers who reviewed 14 years of black tea studies. Not only does black tea hydrate you as well as water does, but it keeps your heart and teeth healthy and improves your mood and alertness.

Research also makes clear the antioxidant power of tea. Scientists at Tufts University in Boston compared the "ORAC" capacity of tea with that of 22 vegetables. ORAC refers to the Oxygen Radical Absorbance Capacity, a measurement of the total antioxidant power of foods and other chemical substances: The higher the ORAC score, the greater its antioxidant capacity. Although there was variation among various teas, the highest scoring teas were green tea and black tea, brewed for 5 minutes. They outranked the best fruits and vegetables.

And Greek researchers concluded in a recent study that drinking tea is linked to lower blood sugar among healthy senior citizens.

||||||||||||||||||||||||||||||||||||||||||||||

Tea 101

All non-herbal tea is made from the same plant. So what makes for the different types of tea? How it is processed.

To make **black** tea, the dried leaves are crushed to liberate enzymes, which react with the catechins over a few hours to produce changes in color and flavor. This is often referred to as "fermentation." **Green** tea is not fermented; the leaves are first steamed to halt any enzyme activity. **Oolong** tea is partially fermented.

on the horizon

In late 2009, scientists from the Boston Biomedical Research Institute and the University of Pennsylvania announced a breakthrough that could potentially change the prognosis of fatal brain disorders like Alzheimer's, Huntington's, and Parkinson's diseases. They found that when they combined the green tea component EGCG with another chemical called DAPH-12, the combo destroyed amyloids, the protein structures that cause these diseases.

Amyloids wrap around brain tissues or fill nerve cells. Eventually, they suffocate the cells and cause loss of memory, language, motor function, and premature death. This study marks the first time scientists have successfully destroyed amyloids, which are notoriously impenetrable structures, the researchers said. Though the findings are cause for hope, they

Herbal teas

These are teas made from the dried leaves of flowers and herbs. While they have entirely different chemical profiles from black or green tea, they still offer many health benefits. Here's a rundown:

Lavender. This tea with a floral bouquet is brewed from dried lavender flowers and can calm you at the end of the day.

Lemon balm. This minty, lemony tea helps soothe jittery nerves.

Nettle. Made from the same plant that causes stinging skin irritation, nettle tea is rich in vitamin C and several minerals. Herbalists recommend it to treat arthritis, allergic rhinitis, and gout and to increase milk production in nursing mothers. Avoid it during pregnancy because it may cause uterine contractions.

Peppermint. Tea from this mint plant is refreshing (especially iced in the summer). It stimulates digestion and dispels gas. Avoid it if you have a hiatal hernia because peppermint promotes reflux of the stomach contents into the esophagus.

Raspberry leaf. Herbalists recommend raspberry tea to ease menstrual cramps.

Rose hips. Rich in vitamin C, rose hips tea can serve as an alternative to orange juice.

Rosemary. Tea from this popular garden herb can boost memory and alertness, but drinking more than two or three cups a day may irritate the stomach.

Rooibos. The leaves of Southern Africa's rooibos (pronounced roy-boss) plant (*Aspalathus linearis*) have been brewed as a refreshing beverage for centuries. Its delicious flavor and remarkable antioxidant capacity gives it the potential to improve general health and well-being.

Sage. A cup of sage tea before bedtime may prevent menopausal night sweats.

Thyme. Herbalists recommend thyme tea for gastrointestinal complaints and especially to treat lung congestion and coughs.

are still extremely preliminary. Next steps for the researchers will be to further explore the EGCG combination and its potential against these dreaded diseases.

green tea and cancer

Researchers suspect that polyphenols in green tea may play an important role in cancer prevention—they believe that polyphenols help kill cancer cells and stop their progression.

Recent studies examining green tea's ability to slow prostate, esophageal, and colorectal cancers have posted positive results. In a study of 472 women with breast cancer, those who drank the most green tea experienced the least spread of the disease. They also found that women in the early stages of breast cancer who drank at least five cups of green tea every day before their diagnoses were less likely to have the disease recur after they completed treatment. However, drinking green tea had no effect on women in the late stages of breast cancer.

In skin-cancer studies, lab animals that were given tea developed one-tenth as many tumors as animals that were given water.

While tea is mainly valued for its cancer-preventing powers, there's some evidence that it many help people who already have cancer. The EGCG in green tea inhibits the production of urokinase, an enzyme that cancer cells need in order to grow. It also seems to stimulate the process of programmed cell death, or apoptosis, in cancer cells.

BUYER'S tip

For the freshest tea, shop at a store that has a good turnover rate and buy only as much as you can use in a month. Tea is best stored in a cool, dry pantry. Refrigerating or freezing can ruin its flavor. Green tea has less caffeine than black tea, but otherwise has a similar chemical profile.

Good to Know

Two to three cups of tea a day is probably enough to provide most of the health benefits. One caveat: If you usually take your tea with milk, you might be missing out on some of the health protection. Proteins in milk may bind to tea's polyphenols and block their beneficial effects. If you're sensitive to caffeine, stick with decaf varieties.

thyme

The same herb that adds savor to sauces, soups, stuffings, stews, and salads also makes a handy and effective home remedy for coughs. Thyme is a potent germ-killer that's been approved in Germany for bronchitis, whooping cough, and upper respiratory infections. When diluted, its essential oil can help prevent gum disease and athlete's foot. And here's something we bet you didn't know: Thyme tea can neutralize foul-smelling flatulence.

rooted in history

Ancient Sumerians and Egyptians used thyme (*Thymus vulgaris*) as a medicine and also to embalm the dead, which we hope says more about thyme's preservative powers than its medicinal ones. The Romans believed that bathing in thyme would provide vigor; they also burned it to repel venomous creatures and made thyme-infused cheese and even alcoholic beverages. As early as the 1600s, British herbalist Nicholas Culpeper recognized thyme's ability to treat coughs and called it "a noble strengthener of the lungs." He wrote that thyme was the best treatment for "hooping cough," purging phlegm, and relieving shortness of breath.

Thyme was one of the first herbs European settlers brought to the New World, and colonists grew it in their gardens. They brewed thyme tea to relieve cold symptoms, including fever, congestion, cough, and disturbed sleep.

Thyme's main constituent, thymol, is a strong anti-septic, which prompted Missourian Joseph Lawrence to include it in the mouthwash he invented in 1879, which he called Listerine.

what's in it?

Thymol, thyme's most abundant medicinal constituent, kills *Porphyromomas gingivalis*, *Selenomonas artemidis*, and *Streptococcus sobrinus*, which are common germs associated with periodontal disease, tooth decay, and oral infections. Thyme also contains flavonoids that prevent muscle spasms as well as rosmarinic acid, an antioxidant that helps reduce inflammation.

thyme fights coughs

Thyme's expectorant, antiseptic, and antispasmodic properties suppress coughs, loosen congestion, and fight infections in the throat and lungs. Another reason for thyme's effectiveness as a cough and congestion remedy is that thyme oil, when ingested, is removed from the body through the lungs. As a result, its healing constituents can work directly where they are most needed.

BUYER'S tip

Find dried thyme leaves in the spice section of the super-market. Thyme comes in many varieties and makes a wonderful, low-growing garden herb. Lemon thyme is especially attractive and tasty.

Good to Know

While all culinary usages of thyme are perfectly healthy and safe, don't take thyme medicinally during pregnancy (culinary amounts are fine). Never take pure thyme oil internally. Dilute thyme essential oil in a carrier oil such as olive oil before using it externally because pure thyme oil can irritate skin.

turmeric

Turmeric (*Curcuma longa*) might well be the most promising of all the medicinal herbs. You know it as the citrusy-sharp spice that gives a golden glow to curry. But over the last decade or so, medical researchers have focused serious attention on turmeric. In particular, they're interested in a component of the herb called curcumin, a potent antioxidant that dramatically reduces inflammation. Studies also show that curcumin has a protective effect on the liver. What's more, recent research reveals it has a remarkable range of potential anticancer effects.

rooted in history

Indians have used turmeric for at least 2,500 years, first as a dye and later as a seasoning. By 700 AD, traders carried it to China and later to Africa. Marco Polo wrote about turmeric in the 13th century, amazed by the common plant whose rhizome flavored and colored food almost as well as saffron, which was wildly expensive in comparison. An ointment containing turmeric, which was recommended for food poisoning, was mentioned in an Ayurvedic medicine book dating back to 250 BC.

what's in it?

Turmeric's medicinal properties come largely from curcumin and a volatile oil called turmerone. Turmeric also contains more than two dozen anti-inflammatory compounds, including six different COX-2 inhibitors. These

USE FOR

Alzheimer's disease

Arthritis

Asthma

Boils

Bursitis and
  tendinitis

Cancer prevention

Eczema

High cholesterol

Memory

Psoriasis

Ringworm

compounds inhibit the COX-2 enzyme, which speeds up the formation of substances that cause inflammation and pain and may also cause tumor cells to grow. Turmeric also contains compounds that block the formation of beta-amyloid, the substance responsible for the plaques that diminish brain function and cause Alzheimer's disease.

what science says

Biochemists at the University of Illinois at Urbana-Champaign recently made a landmark discovery about how the body regulates inflammation. In a nutshell, they deciphered a molecular code that controls the function of a protein called NF-kappa B. This protein acts like a molecular "switch" that flips on when the cell is under attack and off when the attack has been cleared. When switched on, NF-kappa B moves into the cell's nucleus and triggers the proteins that cause inflammation. When the switch doesn't get turned off, which can happen when the cell is under stress, "things can go crazy in the body," said the researchers.

What does all this biochemistry have to do with turmeric? Good question. Turns out, turmeric plays a role in turning off NF-kappa B, says a leading researcher from the University of Texas MD Anderson Cancer Center in Houston. Taking 1 teaspoon (2 g) of turmeric a day can lessen the effects of inflammatory conditions, such as rheumatoid arthritis, osteoarthritis, asthma, and, potentially, cancer, heart disease, diabetes, and depression.

Separately, turmeric has been shown to reduce harmful cholesterol levels in the blood and reduce the development of hardened and blocked arteries. Clinical trials also have shown turmeric is effective in reducing the symptoms of rheumatoid arthritis and postoperative inflammation.

on the horizon

Researchers began investigating turmeric's potential against cancer when they noticed that some studies showed that people living in India, where turmeric is a key ingredient in many recipes, had up to a 50 percent lower incidence of cancer. Subsequent test tube and animal studies have confirmed that curcumin kills cancer cells and slows tumor growth. But much more study is needed before we know whether or not curcumin can become an effective cancer treatment.

BUYER'S tip

India produces nearly all the world's turmeric, and as it turns out, also consumes 80 percent of the crop, according to reports. That said, turmeric is easy to find: It will be in the spice aisle of any major supermarket. It should be a bright marigold color and have lots of fragrance. Keep it well sealed and store in a cool, dry, dark pantry.

Good to Know

Use only in culinary amounts during pregnancy. High medicinal doses may inhibit fertility. Don't take large doses if you take anticoagulants or non-steroidal anti-inflammatory drugs (NSAIDs).

vinegar

Its name comes from the French word *vinaigre*, or "sour wine," and it's a mouth-puckering liquid that not only puts the zing in your salad but is also the bane of bacteria, the foe of fungi, the solution to jellyfish stings, and the soother of sunburns. In fact, over the past 5,000 years, vinegar has taken aim against everything from headaches and sore muscles to the Black Death. Used correctly, it can settle your stomach, stave off swimmer's ear, make hair more lustrous, and soften skin. Some people swear that vinegar mixed with honey and warm water can take the pain out of leg cramps. Others use vinegar to dry up cold sores. What's more, it's an antiseptic "green cleaner" that shines glass as well as high-priced cleaning sprays. Hard to believe that something so sour can be so sweet for your health!

rooted in history

Back in 5000 BC, the Babylonians turned date palm fruit into vinegar and used it to pickle and preserve foods. From residue found in ancient urns, we know that the Egyptians were also using vinegar, probably for similar reasons, around 3000 BC. Vinegar is mentioned in both the Old and New Testaments of the Bible: In Ruth 2:14 is a passage about Ruth dipping bread into vinegar to refresh herself after slaving in the barley fields. Hippocrates, the Greek father of medicine, prescribed vinegar mixed with honey to treat ills including coughs and colds.

USE FOR

Acne

Athlete's foot

Body odor

Bruises

Calluses and corns

Dandruff

Diarrhea

Digestive problems

Ear infections

Fatigue

Foot problems

Head lice

Healthy skin
  and teeth

Hemorrhoids

Hives

Insect bites

Jock itch

Nosebleed

Oily hair

Sinusitis

Sore throat

Sunburn

In World War I, soldiers' wounds were bathed in vinegar, and even today, if you can stand the sting, it's an adequate disinfectant if you have a scratch or sore.

what's in it?

Vinegar can be made from a huge number of plants, but all have one thing in common. Put a drop of vinegar—any type—on your tongue, and you'll know immediately what gives the tangy liquid its puckery nature. Vinegar is acidic, thanks to a high concentration of acetic acid, formed when bacteria feast on a fermented liquid. Acetic acid kills bacteria and fungi and is the active ingredient in some drugs that treat ear infections.

vinegar for weight loss

Japanese scientists reported in a recently completed study that when mice were fed a high-fat diet and given vinegar supplements, they developed about 10 percent less body fat than mice that got only the fatty food. They discovered that vinegar worked at a genetic level by influencing genes linked to fatty acid oxidation and energy-burning proteins. The scientists believe that vinegar suppresses body fat accumulation, though more studies are needed to see whether vinegar can have the same effect in people.

Good to Know

Too much vinegar may cause stomach upset. People who are allergic to molds may develop a reaction to non-distilled vinegar.

BUYER'S tip

Healers tend to prefer apple cider vinegar for use in home remedies. Here's why: Fermented apples are rich in pectin, a type of fiber that's excellent for digestion. Apples also contain malic acid, which combines with magnesium in your body to help fight aches and pains. So unless told otherwise, use cider vinegar for healing.

Around the world with vinegar

Wherever you travel, you'll find native varieties of vinegar brewed from whatever is locally handy. In the Philippines, it's sugarcane; in Thailand, it's coconut; and in China, red, white, and black rice wine vinegars have flavored stir-fries for more than 5,000 years.

Elsewhere you'll find vinegar made from honey, potatoes, dates, nuts, and berries. And in the Mediterranean, it's grapes that become red and white wine vinegars. Americans are most familiar with cider vinegar (from apples) or plain, distilled white vinegar that's the product of grain.

wheat germ

USE FOR

Allergies

Asthma

Blood sugar stabilization

Breast tenderness

Dry skin

Heart health

High cholesterol

Hot flashes

Improved immunity

Menstrual symptoms

Stress

Warts

Wheat germ is the nutritional heart of the wheat kernel. When white flour is processed, this "germ" is milled out; that's why white flour contains so little nutritive value. Although it's the smallest part of the grain, the germ is chock-full of nutrients, including vitamin E, thiamine, folate, magnesium, and zinc. It's also one of the few plant parts in nature that contains the entire vitamin B-complex.

rooted in history

Wheat is one of man's longest-cultivated grains and has been farmed for as long as 9,000 years. Wheat became an ancient symbol of prosperity, fertility, abundance, and life. The fertility gods of Greece, Egypt, and Rome shared wheat as one of their symbols. Native Americans cultivated wheat, baking it into breads, tortillas, and cakes, and brewing it into beverages.

In Ayurveda, the traditional medical system of India, wheat is used to treat stress and mental problems and is said to strengthen the muscles.

what's in it?

The vitamin E in wheat germ contains a powerful anti-oxidant that is linked to heart health as well as a strong immune system. The fat in wheat germ (1.5 g in 2 table-spoons) is predominantly polyunsaturated fat, which can help lower LDL cholesterol levels when it replaces saturated fat in the diet. Wheat germ is also a source of plant sterols that help lower cholesterol levels.

And because it is a complex carb that is slow to digest, wheat germ has a low glycemic index (GI) number and may reduce the risk of type-2 diabetes. According to a recent study by Harvard Medical School, eating more whole-grain foods, such as wheat germ, reduces the risk of type 2 diabetes for women.

Good to Know

Whenever you can, include a little of this delicious whole grain when you're cooking or baking. Its nutty flavor enhances banana or zucchini bread, rice pudding, coffee cake, apple crisp, pizza dough, bread dough, savory pie dough, and even homemade cookies. You can sprinkle it over cereals or on top of salads, mix it into meat loaf, hamburgers, or veggie burgers, or use it as a substitute for some or all of the bread crumbs when coating fish, chicken, or vegetables.

BUYER'S tip

Find wheat germ in the cereal aisle of your supermarket and in health food stores. Wheat germ is sold in both toasted and natural forms. Once it has been opened, keep the wheat germ jar tightly sealed and refrigerated to prevent it from going rancid. Defatted wheat germ contains much less vitamin E and does not need refrigeration. It can be kept in the cupboard.

looking & feeling great

Use your kitchen pantry to boost your appearance and your health

Take a good look around a drugstore, and you quickly realize that medicine takes up only a small amount of the shelf space. Gobbling up much of the real estate are shampoos, skin creams, cosmetics, and other products that aren't meant to make you *feel* better, but rather *look* better.

There's nothing vain about that. Looking your best is a crucial part of being happy, which in turn is a crucial part of good health. Only trouble is, a multibillion-dollar "personal care" industry has us convinced that it takes costly concoctions to achieve that look-good, feel-good balance we all want.

Don't be deceived. Long before the rise of supermodels and mega-beauty brands, our grandparents and their forebears took care of themselves just fine with everyday pantry items. In the pages ahead, you'll find surprising yet effective ways to harness your kitchen pantry to achieve all that you dream of for your health and appearance. And you'll save a fortune achieving it. Now *that's* a beautiful thing.

healthy, smooth skin

You know what healthy skin looks like. It sparkles, no matter how old you are. Even if you haven't inherited a flawless complexion, you can make the most of what you've got without resorting to beauty products whose prices make you weak in the knees. Here's a little secret about some of those expensive products: Many contain ingredients whose effective stand-ins already live on the shelves of your kitchen cabinet.

Skin care basics

Before you embark on a do-it-yourself skin care regimen, it's important to know your skin type and how best to care for it. Skin experts classify complexions into four general types: normal, dry, oily, and sensitive. They also recognize that mature skin requires special care as women transition through menopause and beyond.

Normal skin is clear, supple, and soft, neither too dry nor too oily. It is not overly sensitive to sun, climate, or the environment.

Dry skin looks dull, feels tight after washing, and needs constant protection and moisturizing to avoid flaking and peeling.

Oily skin might feel soft and supple, but it looks shiny and needs to be cleansed several times a day. Pores are larger than those of either normal or dry skin. This type of skin is often prone to blackheads and pimples.

Pantry HEALERS

Almonds

Aloe vera gel

Bay leaves

Chamomile tea

Cinnamon

Cloves

Flaxseeds

Ginger

Green tea

Honey

Lavender
  essential oil

Oats

Olive oil

Peppermint

Rice

Rosemary

Salts

Tea tree oil

Wheat germ

Witch hazel

Sensitive skin reacts badly to sunlight or irritants. It burns easily and may develop rashes, blotches, or spots when exposed to new substances, such as the chemicals often found in commercial skin-cleansing products.

Most people have a combination of skin types—for example, basically normal with some oily areas on the forehead, around the nose, and on the chin, and maybe some dryness around the eyes.

All skin types benefit when you cleanse, tone, and moisturize twice a day—once in the morning and again before bedtime. In addition, two simple DIY treatments—steaming and exfoliating—can help make your skin look spa-pampered.

• *Cleansing:* Choose a cleanser based on your skin type, and perform this essential daily ritual gently to remove makeup and grime.

• *Toning:* After cleansing, use a toner to remove cleanser residue and close the pores.

• *Moisturizing:* Based on your skin type, choose an appropriate moisturizer and smooth over face, neck, and décolletage twice a day.

• *Steaming:* Once or twice a week, give your face a 10-minute steam cleaning. Steaming works naturally to improve microcirculation to the skin's surface. It also flushes out toxins and debris by opening pores and makes

||||||||||||||||||||||||||||||||||||||||||||||||||||||||||||||||||||||||||||||||||||||||||||||||||||||||||||||

Pantry foods for clear skin

Tweaking an unhealthy diet is the first step to enhancing your skin's health and radiance. First move: Cut way back on fatty and sugary foods. These contribute to the inflammation that can worsen any skin condition. Replace unhealthy junk foods with delicious foods rich in antioxidants and other nutrients that are proven to improve skin health. When you keep your larder full of foods like these, you can whip up a healthy snack or meal in less time than it takes to zip through the drive-through. Enjoy them regularly as noted, and your skin will soon reap the rewards.

FOOD	HOW MUCH
Canned salmon	3.5 ounces twice a week
Green tea	2 or more cups a day, hot or iced
Flaxseeds	2 tablespoons freshly ground seeds a day
Olive oil	1 tablespoon a day
Canned sardines	2 ounces once or twice a week
Canola oil	1 tablespoon a day
Brazil nuts	Small handful two or three a times week

it easier for your skin to absorb the essential oils and aromatic herbs in the water.

• *Exfoliating:* Once a week, go over the skin with a simple, homemade scrub blend. This will remove dead skin cells, promote circulation, and improve clarity and radiance.

recipes for cleansing

Fragrant Facial Cleanser

This beautifully scented cleanser is a gentle way to remove makeup and cleanse your skin. It's suitable for all skin types. Almond, jojoba, and avocado oils are light and especially suited for complexion care. You can find them at health and natural food stores. If you don't use them, you can substitute olive or canola oil.

> ¼ cup olive oil
> ¼ cup almond, jojoba, or avocado oil (optional)
> 10 drops lavender essential oil

Place the olive oil, almond oil, and lavender oil in a 4-ounce sterilized glass jar with a tight-fitting lid and shake until blended. Store in a cool, dark place. To use, saturate a cotton ball with oil and sweep over your face to remove makeup. Rinse well with warm water and follow with a toner.

Canola–Tea Tree Oil Cleanser

Use this cleanser on normal to dry skin that's prone to the occasional blemish.

> ¼ cup canola oil
> 10 drops tea tree oil

Place the canola oil and tea tree oil in a 4-ounce sterilized glass jar with a tight-fitting lid and shake until blended. Store in a cool, dark place. To use, saturate a cotton ball with oil and sweep over your face to remove makeup. Rinse well with warm water and follow with a toner.

recipes for toning

Clarifying Green Tea Toner

This gently astringent blend contains vinegar to restore the skin's pH balance. The anti-oxidant-rich green tea helps counter sun damage, while the fennel seeds are said to be cleansing and hydrating. You can find vegetable glycerin at health food stores and online.

    1 tablespoon green tea leaves (cut open a tea bag or two)
    1 teaspoon crushed fennel seeds
    ½ cup boiling water
    2 tablespoons apple cider vinegar
    1 teaspoon vegetable glycerin

1. Place the tea leaves and fennel seeds in a bowl and cover with the boiling water. Cover the bowl and allow the herbs to steep until the water cools. Strain. Combine the fennel water, vinegar, and glycerin in a bottle.

2. To use, shake well. Saturate a cotton ball with the liquid and wipe over your skin after cleansing. Store the toner in the refrigerator and use within 10 days.

Minty Astringent

Barley water is a good source of zinc and sulfur, two minerals that help balance oil production. Peppermint is refreshing and stimulating, and rosemary calms inflammation.

    1 tablespoon dried peppermint
    1 tablespoon dried rosemary
    ½ cup witch hazel
    2 tablespoons vodka
    1 tablespoon pearl barley
    ½ cup water
    5 drops peppermint essential oil (optional)

1. Grind the peppermint and rosemary in a blender or clean coffee grinder. Transfer to a jar with a tight-fitting lid.

2. Add the witch hazel and vodka. Cover the jar tightly and shake vigorously for a few minutes. Put the jar in the pantry and steep for 10 days. After 10 days, strain the liquid into a sterilized canning jar with a tight-fitting lid.

3. Put the barley in a saucepan with the water. Bring to a boil, then reduce the heat and simmer, covered, for 15 minutes. Cool, then strain, reserving liquid.

4. Combine the barley water and herbal liquid in a bottle. Add the peppermint oil, if using.

5. Shake well before each use. Store in the refrigerator for up to two weeks. Apply to skin with a cotton pad.

Aromatherapy Skin Spritz

Use this instant refresher to remove cleanser residue and excess perspiration and oil, especially during hot weather. Grapefruit and lemon oils have gentle astringent and bleaching properties, while apple cider vinegar balances the skin's pH.

½ cup carbonated mineral water
½ cup witch hazel
1 tablespoon apple cider vinegar
5 drops lavender essential oil
5 drops grapefruit essential oil
3 drops lemon essential oil

1. Place the water, witch hazel, and vinegar in a pump-spray bottle with a fine mist head. Add the lavender, grapefruit, and lemon oils.

2. To use, shake and lightly spritz over the face and neck, avoiding eyes. Store in the refrigerator for up to one month.

 recipes for moisturizing

Daily Moisturizer

This moisturizer will leave your complexion moist and replenished and is perfect for normal or combination skin. Smooth on twice a day after toning. You can substitute virgin olive oil for the apricot kernel, jojoba, and wheat germ oils (available at any health food store), but the result won't be quite as light or nourishing.

2 tablespoons apricot kernel oil
1 teaspoon jojoba oil
1 teaspoon wheat germ oil
6 drops lavender essential oil
2 drops lemon essential oil (omit if using on sensitive skin)

Place all the ingredients in a sterilized glass jar with a tight-fitting lid and shake well. Store in a cool, dark place and use within two months.

Don't forget the sunscreen!

Many commercial moisturizers have built-in sunscreens, but homemade recipes don't. Remember to use sunscreen of at least 15 SPF or higher whenever you're outside in the sun.

healthy nails

Well-groomed fingernails make a great first impression. But brittle, flaking nails or cracked, dry cuticles do not. As for toenail fungus, well, it can make you want to stash your sexy sandals in the closet. If you tend to hide your nails from sight, you'll be happy to discover these simple remedies. They all come straight from your kitchen cabinet and can make your nails so healthy and attractive that you'll want to show them off for all to see.

kitchen cabinet cures

Slather hands and cuticles. Frequent applications of moisturizer prevent scraggy-looking cuticles and brittle nails. Keep hand lotion handy in several key places: beside the kitchen sink, near the tub or shower, in your purse or car, next to your favorite chair, in your desk drawer, and on your nightstand. Hiding lotion in plain sight will help you remember to slather it on several times a day.

Enrich nails from within. If your nails are brittle or flaking, try getting more essential omega-3 fatty acids in your diet. These are found in foods such as canned fatty fish, nuts, freshly ground flaxseeds, and flaxseed oil. Just a few servings per week of canned salmon, sardines, or mackerel can put you on the path to healthier nails. If you don't eat much fish, take 1 tablespoon flaxseed oil a day (use it in place of other oil in salad dressing), or sprinkle 2 tablespoons freshly ground flaxseeds on your cereal or other food every day.

Pantry HEALERS

Avocado oil

Canned fatty fish

Epsom salts

Flaxseed oil

Flaxseeds

Jojoba oil

Lavender
 essential oil

Moisturizer

Olive oil

Petroleum jelly

Tea tree oil

Thyme

When to call THE DOCTOR

Unless you suspect you have an underlying nutritional deficiency, nail problems are generally cosmetic problems, not health issues. As for nail fungus, it's tenacious and can take months or even years to clear up on its own. If the two-step soak and tea tree treatment doesn't clear up the problem after at least three months of diligent, regular use, consult your doctor to discuss options.

Do this before bedtime. For dry or brittle nails, rub petroleum jelly or olive oil into your nails to hold moisture around and under your nails. Then, slip a pair of thin cotton gloves on your hands before you to sleep.

Sooth ingrown toenails. If you don't clip your nails straight across, or if your shoes don't fit properly, you can wind up with a painful ingrown toenail. Here's a soothing treatment: Fill a 5-gallon bucket with about 2 gallons of hot water. Add a handful of Epsom salts and stir until the salt dissolves. Soak your problem foot for 15 to 20 minutes each day. Hot water softens the skin around the ingrown nail while the Epsom salts will combat infection and reduce swelling.

Treat toenail fungus with tea tree oil. Applying 100 percent tea tree oil for a minimum of three months has been shown to kill nail fungus as well as a prescription antifungal cream. In the study, 60 percent of both groups completely or partially eradicated their symptoms. Once or twice a day—every day—apply a drop or two of tea tree oil to the discolored nail. Be careful not to apply tea tree to the skin because undiluted tea tree oil may be irritating. Make sure to use 100 percent pure tea tree essential oil; products that only contain a little oil won't work.

Nail no-no's

Quick-drying nail polishes: They may save time, but at the expense of your nails. Most of these formulas contain more formaldehyde and alcohol than regular polishes, both of which are drying and make nails prone to splitting. To fast-dry nails naturally, do this: Fill your bathroom sink part way with ice cubes, then fill with cold water. After each coat of nail polish, dip your wet nails into the cold water for a minute or two. Miraculously, they'll be dry when you take them out.

Artificial nails: They can seem like a godsend to women who have problems with weak, soft, brittle nails, and for women who bite or pick at their nails. Trouble is, fake nails can breed fungus. What's more, when artificial nails are glued on top of your real ones, the gap in between creates a breeding ground in which you can develop a painful bacterial infection. So forgo the fakes, no matter how much you long for elegant nails.

recipes for healthy nails

Rich Aromatherapy Cuticle Oil

The essential oils in this rich, softening blend help to counter cracked and ragged cuticles. Tea tree oil is a proven fungus fighter, while lavender is anti-inflammatory and healing. You can find avocado and jojoba oil in health food stores, or you can substitute olive oil for either or both.

> 1 tablespoon jojoba oil
> 1 tablespoon avocado oil
> 10 drops tea tree essential oil
> 10 drops lavender essential oil

1. Pour the jojoba and avocado oils into a small, dark-colored glass bottle, which will help preserve the oil.
2. Add the tea tree and lavender essential oils, screw on cap, and shake to combine.
3. Before using the cuticle oil, shake the bottle well, then massage a few drops into your nails and cuticles daily to soften your cuticles and prevent them from splitting.

Double-Powered Nail Fungus Treatment

Thyme and tea tree oil annihilate fungal infections; lavender is soothing and healing. Use this soak several times a week, then follow with the aromatherapy oil regimen in the previous recipe. The key to this treatment is regularity and patience: You have to use this double-barrel treatment regularly for at least three months in order to send fungus packing.

> 2 teaspoons dried thyme
> 10 drops tea tree essential oil
> 10 drop lavender essential oil

Steep the thyme, covered, in 1 cup of boiling water for 15 minutes before straining. Allow to cool and then swirl in the tea tree and lavender essential oils. Soak affected nails in the liquid for 15 minutes twice a day.

healthy teeth & mouth

When your teeth and gums are in tip-top shape, it's not just your appearance that benefits. Heart disease, diabetes, pneumonia, and even chronic lung disease are all linked to unhealthy gums. Researchers suspect that as bacteria from your gums travel throughout your bloodstream, they create low-level inflammation that can trigger or promote a variety of chronic diseases. Happily, effective and economical natural remedies for a sparkling smile and a healthy, sweet-smelling mouth are as close as your kitchen pantry.

kitchen cabinet cures

Stock xylitol gum and mints. This natural sugar alcohol (found in berries, vegetables, mushrooms, and birch trees) may look and taste just like sugar, but there's where the resemblance ends. Xylitol contains 40 percent fewer calories than sugar, and quite unlike sugar, it prevents cavities and plaque formation by inhibiting the growth of decay-promoting bacteria. A report published in the *Journal of the American Dental Association* said that chewing xylitol gum for five minutes after eating, three to five times a day, inhibits plaque accumulation and prevents cavities. And just recently, a team of Japanese dentists discovered that when pregnant women began chewing xylitol gum in their sixth month of pregnancy and continued using the gum for a year, their babies were much less likely to develop cavity-causing bacteria compared to pregnant women who didn't chew the gum. Look for gums or mints labeled "all xylitol" or those containing xylitol as the only sweetener.

Be a tea drinker. Flavonoids and other tea ingredients seem to prevent harmful bacteria from sticking to teeth and also block production of a type of sugar that contributes to cavities. Tea also contains high amounts of fluoride. Alternate between green and black tea and enjoy a few cups a day.

Gargle with apple cider vinegar in the morning. The vinegar helps remove stains, whiten teeth, and kill bacteria in your mouth and gums. Brush as usual after you gargle.

Brush your teeth with baking soda once a week. This will help remove stains and whiten your teeth. Use it just as you would toothpaste. You can also use salt as an alternative toothpaste. If your gums start to feel raw, switch to brushing with salt every other day.

Chew cinnamon gum once a day. Researchers at the University of Illinois at Chicago have found that cinnamon-flavored chewing gum reduces bacteria in the mouth that cause bad breath. The reason? The gum contains cinnamic aldehyde, an essential oil that inhibits the growth of bacteria responsible for cavities and periodontal infections. Actually, any kind of sugar-free gum chewed after meals will help remove food particles and wash away bacteria because it generates extra saliva.

Some chewing gums actually help prevent cavities and plaque build-up.

recipes for a healthier mouth

Cinnamon Tooth Powder
This easy-to-make recipe polishes and whitens teeth and leaves your mouth feeling super-clean. Cinnamon has antibacterial properties, while clove is both antiseptic and healing.

    2 tablespoons baking soda
    1 teaspoon fine sea salt
    ½ teaspoon powdered cinnamon
    5 drops clove essential oil
    3 drops peppermint essential oil

1. Sift the baking soda, salt, and cinnamon together into a bowl to remove lumps. Add the clove and peppermint oils, then sift again. Store the powder in an airtight container.

2. To use, dampen your toothbrush, dip it in the powder, and brush as you would with toothpaste.

Minty Mouthwash

Cooling peppermint sweetens bad breath and makes your mouth feel clean. Tea tree essential oil fights gum disease, and aloe vera soothes oral tissue.

> 2 peppermint tea bags
> ¾ cup boiling water
> 1 tablespoon fresh aloe gel
> 5 drops tea tree essential oil
> 3 drops peppermint essential oil

1. Place the tea bags in a small glass bowl and cover with the boiling water. Cover the bowl and steep for 30 minutes. Squeeze and remove the tea bags.
2. Add the aloe gel and tea tree and peppermint oils. Mix well. Store in a dark glass container.
3. Shake well, then swish 1 to 2 tablespoons around your mouth, and spit it out. Do not swallow. Store in a cool place and use within one week.

Mouthwash for Bleeding Gums

See your dentist if your gums bleed whenever you brush your teeth. Once you've ruled out any dental problems, try this soothing, healing mouthwash. It contains tannin-rich black tea and witch hazel, which have a toning effect on gums. Green tea is an antioxidant. Myrrh has antiseptic and astringent properties, and herbalists praise its powers for healing oral problems.

> 2 black tea bags
> 2 green tea bags
> ¾ cup boiling water
> 1 tablespoon witch hazel
> 5 drops myrrh tincture

1. Place the black and green tea bags in a glass bowl and cover with the boiling water. Cover the bowl and steep for 30 minutes. Strain.
2. Add the witch hazel and myrrh and mix well. Store in a dark glass bottle.
3. To use, shake well and swish 1 to 2 tablespoons around the mouth and spit it out. Do not swallow. Store in a cool place and use within one week.

super-charged immunity

Your immune system is a complex network of cells, tissues, and organs. When operating at peak efficiency, these elements work together in harmony, like a well-conducted orchestra, to ward off attacks by bacteria, viruses, and fungi whose mission is to enter and infect your body. These days, it's more important than ever to keep your immune system in tip-top shape so that you can more effectively repel illnesses from the simple to the serious. In this chapter, you'll discover essential strategies for building and maintaining a powerful immune system. And we'll arm you with tools you can use to ramp up your immunity. Guess where you'll find those tools? By now, you know the answer: They're all in your kitchen cabinet.

first things first

These four key strategies are the places to start to turbocharge your immunity:

Lay off the sweets. And the fatty foods, unhealthy trans fats, and junk-food carbs. All of these dampen a healthy immune system.

Eat farm foods, not factory foods. Unprocessed fruits, vegetables, dairy products, and even lean meats are packed with the nutrients you need for a powerful immune system. Packaged and processed foods not only get stripped of many of those nutrients, but add in chemicals that do you no good.

Pantry HEALERS

Brazil nuts

Canned fatty fish (salmon, sardines)

Dried mushrooms

Farm foods (unprocessed fruits and vegetables, lean meats, dairy products)

Fiber-rich foods

Flaxseeds

Garlic

Green tea

Pumpkin seeds

Raisins

Walnuts

Be active. Exercise is one of the best things you can do to power up immunity. In addition to a brisk 20- to 30-minute walk most days of the week, perform some muscle-building activities at least three times a week. Researchers are learning that muscle mass may help defend against disease-causing microbes—and even help speed recovery from infection and wounds.

Sleep deeply. Right up there with exercise is adequate sleep. Immunity experts say that getting to sleep by 9 or 10 p.m. and resting through the night seems to support immune defense and repair.

kitchen cabinet cures

Scan the shelves for fiber. Think beans, whole-wheat pasta, barley, dried split peas, lentils, nuts, seeds, dried fruits, and whole-grain bread containing 4 grams or more of fiber per serving. Fiber helps lower blood sugar levels and provides immune-enhancing vitamins and minerals.

4 reasons to rethink your drink

That innocent-looking can of soda pop—no matter what it's sweetened with—may be taking a toll on your immunity. Here's why:

1. People who drink sodas instead of healthy beverages (think low-fat milk and pure fruit juice) are less likely to get adequate vitamin A, calcium, and magnesium. What's more, soda contains phosphoric acid that depletes calcium and magnesium. These two nutrients help keep your immunity operating at peak efficiency.

2. Sodas containing high-fructose corn syrup also contain high levels of free radicals linked to tissue damage, the development of diabetes, and diabetic complications.

3. Plastic soda (and water) bottles contain a toxic chemical called bisphenol A (BPA) that can leach from bottles into soda … into you.

Emerging evidence links BPA to myriad maladies, including immune system depression. Public health experts recommend that we protect children from exposure to products containing BPA—especially those they consume or use every day.

4. Diet soda actually *contributes* to weight gain. A study of 1,550 people concluded that people who drink diet soda have a 41 percent increased risk of being overweight or obese—for every can or bottle they drink per day! Turns out, any sweet taste signals body cells to store fat and carbohydrates, which makes you hungrier. Sweet tastes also promote insulin release, which blocks your body's ability to burn fat. The hard truth: No published study has ever proven that drinking diet soda will help you lose weight.

Drink more tea than coffee. Harvard University researchers found that the immune activity of tea drinkers is significantly higher than that of coffee drinkers. They suspect that an amino acid in brewed tea called L-theanine may be involved in tea's immune-enhancing benefits. What's more, green tea is loaded with antioxidants that help damaged cells repair themselves.

Pump some seeds. Yummy pumpkin seeds are rich in zinc, a mineral that's key to a healthy immune system. Studies show that people who are zinc deficient (which is common as we age) have a harder time fending off garden-variety infections. A half cup of pumpkin seeds contains about 6 milligrams of zinc, which is about 40 percent of the recommended daily amount. Calorie alert: If you chow down on delicious, nutritious pumpkin seeds, consider cutting calories elsewhere because ½ cup of pumpkin seeds contains 374 calories.

Samba with selenium. Brazil nuts are packed with the immunity-enhancing antioxidant mineral selenium. Adequate selenium levels enable white blood cells to kill off microbes and tumor cells. Some researchers theorize that because selenium protects cells from free radical damage, a deficiency of the stuff could allow harmless viruses to mutate into more aggressive strains. Once your immune system has been compromised, these more dangerous viruses can then reproduce out of control. They suspect

||||||||||||||||||||||||||||||||||||||||||||||||||||||||||||||||||||||||||||||||||||||||||||||||||||||||||||||||||||||

Vitamin D alert

Are you getting too little of this vital immune-enhancer?

A new groundbreaking study found that nearly 60 percent of the study's participants had too little vitamin D in their blood—and nearly one-quarter of them had serious deficiencies. The study, conducted at the Children's Hospital Los Angeles of the University of Southern California, revealed that low levels of vitamin D put people at risk for a whole spectrum of diseases, including cancer, osteoporosis, diabetes, and autoimmune disorders. What astonished the research team was that the volunteers were healthy, young women living in Southern California, who could logically be expected to benefit from good diets, exercise, and plenty of exposure to sunshine, which triggers the body to produce vitamin D.

Many experts have said that vitamin D's current recommended daily allowance, now set at 400 IU a day, is much too low, and are calling for it to be raised substantially.

Dried mushrooms are packed with nutrients that help prevent disease.

that may be why selenium-deficient HIV patients are far more likely to develop AIDS and die faster. Getting enough selenium rejuvenates immune cells and empowers them to fight germs. Because Brazil nuts contain 75 to 100 micrograms of selenium each, just a couple of nuts a day gives you all the selenium you need. You'll also find selenium in canned salmon (between 34 and 40 micrograms in a 3-ounce portion), raisins, and walnuts.

Glorify the garlic. Rich in antioxidants, especially selenium, garlic can increase production of natural killer cells. Toss chopped or crushed garlic into foods at the very end of cooking, because high temperatures destroy garlic's medicinal action. Better still, use garlic raw whenever possible. For the most potent effect, chop, crush, or cut the cloves 10 to 15 minutes before using and toss directly into salad dressing, sandwich fillings, and other foods.

Opt for omega-3s. Omega-3 fatty acids can strengthen immune function. Omega-3 fatty acids, abundant in cold-water fish, like canned salmon and sardines, as well as in flaxseeds, help reduce acute inflammation, which occurs as part of the immune response to attack or injury. What's more, omega-3s activate parts of the immune system that rein in attack cells to stop them when their job is done.

Get friendly with fungi. Dried mushrooms, including shiitake, maitake, and morels, are packed to the gills with substances that enhance your immunity. Among these are vitamins D, C, K, and the B-complex vitamins riboflavin, niacin, and pantothenic acid. Dried mushrooms are also a rich source of potassium and phosphorous. They're a snap to reconstitute in water, and they add real gourmet flavor to sauces, stews, and casseroles. They last practically forever on the pantry shelf and are usually less expensive than fresh gourmet mushrooms.

stable blood sugar

Do you know what your fasting blood sugar level is? If you don't, you should—especially if you're overweight or have high blood pressure or if diabetes runs in your family. That's because diabetes, the disease that's reaching epidemic proportions in countries all over the world, is marked by elevated blood sugar levels. What's also on the rise? The number of people who have the silent conditions that predict they will someday get diabetes. Researchers now know that diabetes puts you at seriously increased risk for a host of health problems. Among them: heart disease, kidney failure, blindness, infertility, and even cancer. Even if diabetes isn't a concern for you, maintaining blood sugar stability should be. Here's why: Blood sugar levels that spike and dip excessively can trigger mood and energy issues. Help is close at hand if you keep your pantry stocked with weapons to help you win the blood sugar battle.

kitchen cabinet cures

Have a (lunchtime) coffee or two. Recent studies clearly connect coffee drinking with a lower risk for developing diabetes. In one of them, researchers followed the diets of nearly 70,000 nondiabetic French women for about 11 years. During that time, 1,415 of them developed diabetes. Turns out, the women who drank coffee at lunchtime had a significantly lower risk of developing diabetes—and it didn't matter whether they drank regular or decaf.

Pantry HEALERS

Buckwheat flour

Cinnamon

Coffee

Fenugreek

Flaxseeds

High-fiber breads

Soba noodles

Walnuts

Wine

The diabetes epidemic

How widespread has the disease become? Over the past two decades, the number of people worldwide diagnosed with diabetes has gone from 30 million to 246 million. By comparison, in 2008, 33.4 million people worldwide were living with HIV, the virus that causes AIDS. While the diabetes epidemic has been well documented in the United States, it is home to less than 10 percent of the cases worldwide. Seven of the 10 countries with the highest number of diabetics are in the developing world, with China and India leading the way. The World Health Organization conservatively estimates that by 2030, 366 million people worldwide will have diabetes.

These studies build on what researchers already know from at least nine previous studies involving almost 200,000 people in the United States, Europe, and Japan: Coffee drinkers have a substantially lower risk of developing type 2 diabetes.

Do the cinnamon sprinkle. A few years ago, researchers from the U.S. Department of Agriculture studied cinnamon's effects on volunteers with type 2 diabetes. Those who took either 1, 3, or 6 grams of cinnamon (about ½, 1, or 2 teaspoons) or a placebo for 40 days saw their blood glucose levels drop 18 to 29 percent, depending on the amount they took.

More recently, 109 people with poorly controlled diabetes either received standard care, or took ½ teaspoon of cinnamon a day for 90 days (plus standard care). Those who took the cinnamon substantially lowered the critical blood sugar marker, HbA1C. When diabetics lower their HbA1C number to the extent the people in this study did, they lower their risks for developing heart disease by 16 percent, diabetic retinopathy (an eye disease that can cause blindness) by 20 percent, and kidney disease by as much as 33 percent.

Experts suggest that just ½ teaspoon of cinnamon a day can help lower your blood sugar and drop your risks for dangerous diabetic complications. This could be one of the easiest of all home remedies: Just sprinkle this delicious spice into hot and cold cereal, yogurt, coffee, or tea once a day.

Get friendly with fenugreek. If you have prediabetes or type 2 diabetes, meet this little brownish-yellow spice seed. It has a subtle, almost smoky flavor, and it's mostly used in Indian cuisine to flavor curries. Traditional Indian healers use it medicinally for a slew of health problems, including diabetes, and now researchers are discovering that those healers were apparently on the right track. Three different studies have determined that fenugreek lowers glucose levels in type 2 diabetics, increases glycemic control, and decreases insulin resistance. And in a new study, people who took 4 teaspoons of powdered fenugreek every day for eight weeks lowered their fasting blood sugar by 25 percent. They also slashed their triglyceride and LDL (bad) cholesterol numbers, too—by 30 percent each.

To reap fenugreek's blood sugar-lowering benefits, plan to use it daily. You can powder the seeds in a clean coffee grinder and mix with hot water for a tea, or you can mix the powder into breads, muffins, and cooked foods. Aim for 4 teaspoons of powdered fenugreek a day. Do not use fenugreek during pregnancy because it can stimulate uterine contractions.

Stock soba noodles. This tasty Japanese pasta is made from buckwheat flour, which is milled from a fruit seed, so it's not a true grain. In a Canadian study on rats with type 1 diabetes, consuming regular amounts of buckwheat lowered their blood glucose levels by 12 to 19 percent. The study's authors concluded that buckwheat is "a safe, easy, and inexpensive way to lower glucose levels and reduce diabetic complications, including heart, nerve, and kidney problems." In another study, when researchers followed almost 36,000 women in Iowa for six years, they discovered that women who ate three servings of whole grains a day, including buckwheat, had a 21 percent lower risk of diabetes than women who ate just one serving a week. Buckwheat is also a good source of fiber and important minerals. Use buckwheat flour in recipes for pancakes, muffins, and breads.

Choose fiber-rich bread. Search for whole-grain breads that contain at least 3 grams of fiber and 3 grams of protein per slice (more is better). High-fiber whole-grain bread slows the absorption of glucose and decreases insulin spikes. According to the journal *Diabetes Care*, eating whole grains regularly reduces your risk for developing type 2 diabetes.

Enjoy a glass of wine with your dinner. One study found that women who had a drink of wine a day cut their risk of diabetes in half compared to teetotalers. Not a wine lover? The study found the same effects for beer. But cork the wine bottle once dinner is over. An Australian study found that drinking a glass of wine immediately after eating can result in a sudden drop in the insulin in your blood, meaning the glucose from your meal hangs around longer, eventually damaging arteries.

Make some walnut burgers. You'd be surprised how delectable—and easy—it is to use walnuts in recipes for burgers, meatballs, and other tasty treats. And they add a yummy crunch when toasted and tossed into salads. The latest research confirms that eating walnuts is a brilliant strategy for people with type 2 diabetes. In new study

Pantry no-nos

There's more to stable blood sugar than adding certain foods and spices to your diet. Even more important is what you choose not to eat. In general, simple carbohydrates are the foods that most spark blood-sugar surges (and the blood sugar plunges that follow). The reason: Their chemical structure is so simple that they are digested into blood sugar almost instantly. For stable blood sugar—and to help avoid many conditions linked to wild blood-sugar swings— stay away from the following foods, which interestingly tend toward the color white:

- Refined sugar
- High-fructose corn syrup
- White bread
- Pancakes
- White-flour cakes and cookies
- White rice
- White potatoes
- Plain spaghetti
- Corn flakes

Switch to buckwheat pancakes and noodles for flavor and your health.

conducted at Yale University School of Medicine, researchers put 24 people with type 2 diabetes on diets containing a half cup a day of walnuts or on walnut-free diets. After eight weeks, the walnut eaters had significantly improved heart health markers. Separately, Australian researchers recently put 50 overweight type 2 diabetics on one of two diet plans—one group ate a daily quarter-cup serving of walnuts; the other group went walnut-free. After a year, the walnut eaters had significantly greater reductions in their fasting insulin levels.

Since a half cup of walnuts a day contains 327 calories, you'll want to cut an equivalent amount of calories elsewhere in your diet. You can find simple, tasty main-dish walnut recipes online. Not so incidentally, walnuts are an excellent source of omega-3 fatty acids, are proven to lower cholesterol, and even help prevent and control high blood pressure.

Go wild with freshly ground flaxseeds. Their toasty, nutty flavor enhances almost everything you sprinkle them on. Not only do they contain a healthy dose of fiber, they also contain omega-3 fats that help maintain flexible cell membranes. This is critical for people with diabetes, because flexible cell membranes respond to insulin and absorb glucose better. As a result, studies find that flaxseeds may help lower elevated blood sugar. Sprinkle freshly ground flaxseeds over your salad, yogurt, and cereal, for starters. You can also mix them into meatloaf or stir them into pancake and muffin batter.

healthy weight

Obesity absolutely devastates your health. It's linked not only to an increased risk of the problems you'd expect—heart disease and diabetes, as well as joint pain—but also to numerous others you may not consider, such as cancer, hearing loss, Alzheimer's disease, and gastrointestinal problems. Employ these wise kitchen moves, and you're likely to find that achieving your weight-loss goals will become a little bit easier.

kitchen cabinet cures

Portion nuts in snack-sized bags. A study from the City of Hope National Medical Center found that over-weight people who ate a moderate-fat diet containing almonds lost more weight than a control group that didn't eat nuts. Really, any nut will do.

But if you're unaware of how many nuts you're eating, you could end up gaining weight instead of losing it. The appropriate serving size for nuts is 1 ounce, or about 200 calories, depending on the nut. To keep yourself from mindlessly nibbling more than you need, do this: When you buy nuts, open the container and put handful-sized portions into ziplock snack or sandwich bags. And by handful, we mean the amount of nuts you can hold in the palm of your hand with your fingers closed. Then, limit yourself to a serving or two a day.

Pantry HEALERS

Anchovies

Canned fish

Canned soups and
   vegetables

Capers

Cereals

Hot sauces

Lentils

Nonfat powdered
   milk

Nuts

Oatmeal

Seltzer

Soba buckwheat
   noodles

Tea (green or black)

Whole grains
   (instant barley,
   quinoa, tabbouleh)

Whole-wheat pasta

Make 3 smart switches

Just by making these three little dietary tweaks, you could lose 25 pounds in a year.

Skip the sugary drinks. If you drink non-diet soda, you can cut 160 calories (per 16 ounces) out of your day just by switching to a sugar-free quaff. The best beverage choices: green or black tea (hot or iced) or seltzer flavored with a squeeze of lemon or lime, or, of course, just plain water.

Start with soup. Studies show that people who start a meal with soup—especially broth-based soup—end up eating fewer calories by the end of the day without feeling hungrier. Avoid high-calorie cream-based soups and watch the sodium content. Bean soups are especially filling.

Read the labels. Avoid any prepared food that lists sugar, fructose, or corn syrup among the first four ingredients on the label. You should be able to find a lower-sugar version of the same type of food. Also, seek out sugar-free pantry items such as ketchup, mayonnaise, and salad dressing.

Buy the smaller size. It's a fact that the larger the portion in front of you, the more you'll eat. When researchers sent 79 parents home with a movie and either 1- or 2-pound bags of M&Ms along with either a medium or jumbo tub of popcorn for each family member, they ate more M&Ms from the 2-pound bag than from the 1-pound bag and about half a tub of popcorn, regardless of the tub size. Though we're certainly not promoting M&Ms as a weight-loss food (we sincerely wish we could), we do recommend ordering the small bag of popcorn when you're at the movies and buying single-serving–sized snack food packs instead of jumbo sizes. The extra money you might save buying larger sizes isn't worth derailing your weight-control efforts.

Stock these three cans. Canned beans, corn, and tomatoes stretch higher calorie dishes and also combine to make yummy, low-cal meals. Try these great ideas:

• Add a can each of corn, garbanzo beans, and plum tomatoes to your pasta salad recipe. You'll boost the salad's texture and flavor, and as a bonus, you'll be able to eat more salad for just a few more calories. As a double bonus, you'll get healthy amounts of fiber and important nutrients.

• Toss a can of light tuna with a can of white beans. Add a drizzle of olive oil, a squeeze or two of lemon, and a sprinkle of oregano.

• Mix a can of kidney or black beans with a can of corn, and add some canned salsa and a few shots of hot sauce for a tasty lunch.

• Simmer a can of Italian plum tomatoes with a little garlic for a superfast pasta sauce. Serve over 1 cup of whole-wheat pasta.

Pull a caper in your kitchen. You can add oodles of flavor to many foods—for next to no calories—by keeping capers and anchovies in your pantry. Since richly flavored foods are more satisfying than bland foods, you can eat less without feeling deprived. Capers are the tiny pickled buds that give a great zing to bean, tuna, and salmon salads. Rinse before using. And even if you think you don't like anchovies, try adding a few, well-minced, to chicken or tuna salads and tomato sauces. For a delicious low-cal pasta, simmer a large can of Italian plum tomatoes with a can of light tuna, minced garlic, a pinch of dried red pepper flakes, and a few minced anchovies for a few minutes. Serve over whole-wheat pasta. Omega-3 alert: Anchovies are a rich source of this heart-healthy fat.

Use nonfat powdered milk in coffee. You get the nutritional benefits of skim milk, which is high in calcium and low in calories. And powdered milk doesn't dilute coffee the way liquid milk does. And it's far lower in calories and fat than half-and-half.

Eat cereal for breakfast five days a week. Studies find that people who eat cereal for breakfast every day are much less likely to be obese and have diabetes than those who don't. They also take in more vitamins, fiber, and calcium—and less fat—than people who eat other breakfast foods. Of course, that doesn't mean reaching for the ultrasweet kid choices (which is as unhealthy for them as it is for you, by the way). Instead, serve a high-fiber, low-sugar cereal like Kashi GoLean, Total, or Grape-Nuts. To sweeten, add berries (fresh or dried) or sliced banana. And check the package to see what is considered a single portion size. For many dry cereals, a healthy serving is just 1 cup—but many adults pour out at least twice that amount.

Have oatmeal on the weekends. You may not have time on weekday mornings to cook a bowl of oatmeal, so weekends are ideal for enjoying this satisfying, nutrition-rich breakfast. An especially toothsome, stick-to-the-ribs choice is steel-cut Irish oats. Oats are packed with unique compounds, like beta-glucan, which helps lower cholesterol and stabilizes blood sugar, and potent antioxidants called avenanthramides, which reduce heart attack risk. Oats also pack a healthy 4 grams of fiber and just 150 calories per 1-cup serving. Best of all, a bowl of oatmeal keeps you feeling fuller longer, so you're better able to resist food cravings between breakfast and lunch.

Spice it up! Use hot sauce, salsa, cayenne, and Cajun seasonings instead of relying on butter and creamy or sugary sauces. Besides providing lots of flavor with no fat and few calories, many of these spicy seasonings turn up your digestive fires, causing your body to temporarily burn more calories. What's more, capsaicin, the ingredient that puts the fire in hot peppers, can put the chill on your appetite. For a surprising taste treat, sprinkle a little cayenne pepper over air-popped popcorn.

A simple way to eat less

It's a fact that when you serve food on large-sized plates, you tend to load more food on the plate, making it easier to overeat. So switch your dinner-sized plates for smaller lunch-sized plates, and you'll automatically eat less. Need more help controlling portion sizes? Remember the basic rule of portion mix: one-quarter of your plate should hold a lean protein; one-quarter should hold a carbohydrate portion, preferably whole grain; the remaining half should be filled with vegetables.

Pantry HEALERS

Almonds

Broccoli

Canned fish (salmon, sardines, herring, tuna)

Cashews

Coffee

Dried fruit

Leafy greens

Rosemary essential oil

Sage

improved memory

Do you remember the title of the last book you read? Do you scratch your head and wonder whether you've taken your pills this morning? Are names sometimes just beyond your brain's reach? While forgetfulness isn't necessarily a sign that something's wrong, it can be frustrating and sometimes a little scary (especially when you've left that stove burner on…again). Memory boosters and simple do-it-yourself home remedies can help sharpen your memory now and keep it honed for years to come.

kitchen cabinet cures

Make memories with almonds. A recently completed study, conducted by researchers at the Massachusetts Institute of Technology and Tel Aviv University, has revealed just how critical magnesium is for enhancing memory and preventing its impairment. In the study, two groups of elderly rats were given identical diets, but one group was given a magnesium supplement. After testing both groups, the researchers learned the supplement improved the rats' short- and long-term memory and even enhanced their learning ability. The researchers figured out that the number of synapses (nerve endings in the brain that carry memories as electrical impulses) actually increased in the brains of the rats fed the magnesium. But don't race out to the drugstore to pick up bottles of this mineral just yet, warn the researchers. The magnesium supplements currently available don't work the same way as the one the researchers used. The researchers' advice to folks who need a memory boost? Get your magnesium the old-fashioned way, by eating pantry foods like almonds, cashews, and dried fruit. (Leafy greens and broccoli are also super sources.)

Count on coffee. If you drink caffeinated beverages, you'll get a short-term boost in your ability to concentrate. And long-term benefits could be yours as well, especially if you're an older adult. At the Faculty of Medicine in Lisbon, Portugal, researchers concluded that elderly people who drank three or four cups of coffee a day were less likely to experience memory loss than people who drank a cup a day or less. In a French study, women over 80 who drank three cups or more per day were 70 percent less likely to have memory decline than those who drank one cup or less.

Catch a whiff. Buy a little bottle of 100 percent pure rosemary essential oil at the health or natural food store. Tests of brain waves show that inhaling rosemary's aroma increases the brain's production of beta waves, which indicate heightened awareness. Another study showed that inhaling rosemary oil enhanced the memories of test-taking students. To get the memory-boosting benefits, just dab a few drops of the oil on your hair, wrists, clothing, or a handy hankie—anywhere you can get a whiff. Or put some of the oil in a diffuser, and let it fill the air.

Add sage to your cooking. A couple of small studies suggest that the anti-inflammatory effects of sage may boost memory for several hours after eating an extract of the herb. Though those supplements aren't commercially available, you might be able to replicate the results by adding savory sage liberally to various dishes. For example, roast a chicken or turkey with sage-seasoned stuffing; make a tea with 1 teaspoon of the dried herb; use sage in salad dressings and rice dishes; or sprinkle it liberally over pork, poultry, or fish before cooking.

Chow down on tuna or salmon salad. Or enjoy sardines on toast. The same reasons that make canned cold-water fish like salmon, sardines, tuna, and herring so good for your heart also make them good for your brain. The omega-3 oils in fish help "thin" the blood and prevent clogged arteries, and that can keep your brain healthy and, presumably, will help keep your memory sharp.

It's hardly a widespread or accepted form of healing, but there are many people who steadfastly believe that crystals and gems contain a vibrational energy that can help people heal. In fact, gemstone therapy has been around for thousands of years. Proponents note that each stone has its own talent. According to them, amethyst and amber calcite are the gems associated with improved memory. Their message: Carry or wear them everywhere you go, and it will help your mind function more clearly.

easing what ails you

Proven kitchen-cabinet remedies for dozens of the most common health concerns

It wasn't that long ago that huge multi-purpose drugstores didn't exist. Doctors weren't a phone call away, and hospitals and clinics were few and far between. Back in our grandparents' or great-grandparents' day, everyone needed to have at least a smattering of homegrown healing ability to protect their family's health.

And what they learned was how to heal with whatever staples they had on hand. As it turns out, they knew what they were doing. Research confirms that many basic kitchen staples have legitimate, powerful healing properties.

In the pages that follow, we provide hundreds of research-supported pantry cures. Some you'll probably recognize, like using honey to soothe a sore throat. But many others will surprise you—for example, that you can also use Tabasco to help your throat!

Just as importantly, we put these cures in proper perspective. Sometimes, they're all you need to remedy a problem. Other times, they should be used in conjunction with more conventional, doctor-prescribed cures. In all cases, we'll put you on the path toward fast and effective healing.

acne

Even though you're probably long past worrying about your prom-night complexion, acne at any age makes you want to live in a world without mirrors. The umbrella term for the condition in which pores become blocked and often infected, acne causes whiteheads, blackheads, and inflamed skin. Dozens of acne medications are available over the counter and by prescription, but many of them are harsh and can have serious side effects. Fortunately, simple remedies you find in the pantry can often eliminate mild acne—for you and your teenager.

first things first

Keeping your skin clean sounds like pretty obvious advice. But many of us really don't know the very best ways to do that. Here they are:

• Wash body parts where you sprout acne twice a day. Use a mild cleanser, and don't scrub or use exfoliants or facial masks, all of which can make acne worse.

• Keep your hair off your face. When oil from your hair meets oil from your forehead, breakouts may follow. Shampoo every day or two, depending on how oily your hair is, and keep combs, brushes, and anything you use on your hair scrupulously clean.

• Keep your fingers off your face and away from acne. Your hands spread oil, germs, and dirt to everything they touch, even if you can't see dirt on them. Plus scratching, pinching, or rubbing acne can lead to the blemishes getting infected.

• Don't wear a sweatband or tight clothing when you exercise. That can increase your skin's production of oil and lead to both acne and "bacne," those pimples that appear on your shoulders and back.

• If you have severe acne, avoid makeup and lotions. With mild acne, you can use water-based (as opposed to oil-based) makeup. Look for the words "noncomedogenic" or "nonacnegenic" on the label. Wash makeup off your face with soap and water before you go to bed.

kitchen cabinet cures

Dab on tea tree oil. A 5 percent solution of this essential oil from an Australian tree works just as well as the top drugstore acne remedy, benzoyl peroxide, in eradicating pimples, according to Australian researchers. Though tea tree oil doesn't work as quickly as the drugstore cure, it's gentler on your skin. But don't mop it all over your face. It's strong and can dry out your skin, triggering your body to overproduce oil, which can make acne worse. Just dilute a few drops of pure tea tree oil with 20 to 40 drops of witch hazel and apply to skin once or twice a day with a cotton swab. And stay out of the sun—tea tree oil can make you more sensitive to UV rays.

Go clear with green tea. A University of Miami study found that even a mild dose of green tea's antimicrobial and antioxidant compounds erases almost two-thirds of pimples from people with mild to moderate acne when used twice daily for six weeks. But save your money—you don't need to buy the cream. When you whip up a cup of green tea for sipping, whip up a second, let it cool and use it as a face wash, or lay the wet tea bag right on your face like a compress.

Dab on the honey. Honey kills bacteria, which explains why this old folk remedy may improve acne. A particular kind, Manuka honey from New Zealand, is being studied for its antibiotic properties, which are powerful enough to kill methicillin-resistant *Staphylococcus aureus* (MRSA). You don't need to import honey from the other side of the world, though. Just apply a teaspoon of plain honey to affected areas. Some home remedy experts recommend mixing ½ cup of honey into a cup of plain oatmeal, then

When to Call THE DOCTOR

If your blemishes don't respond to natural remedies or over-the-counter medications, you may need some extra help. Contact your doctor if your face becomes seriously inflamed with painful, fluid-filled lumps and a reddish or purplish cast. This could be cystic acne, which can be scarring.

the natural DOCTOR'S Rx

• Switch to organic milk. Because it's hormone-free, it may help decrease acne outbreaks.

• Eat foods rich in antioxidants. Choose a rainbow of brightly colored fruits and vegetables—the more vividly colored, the better.

• Despite the legend, dark chocolate (60 to 70 percent cacao) doesn't promote acne. But, like other sugary and fatty foods, milk chocolate may worsen acne.

Echinacea, the popular herb for colds and immunity, can also help heal acne.

applying the paste to your skin. Leave on for 30 minutes, then rinse. Impurities on the skin adhere to oatmeal and are sloughed away. The oats reduce inflammation and leave a protective barrier on the skin, keeping it moisturized.

Say aloe. This herb, which may be growing on your windowsill right now, fights infection and promotes healing. What's more, applying the gel at least twice a day may reduce scarring. To use, just cut a leaf from the plant, scrape the gel off with a spoon, and apply to affected areas. Or pick up a bottle of 100 percent pure aloe gel at the health food store. Make sure it contains no additional ingredients.

Use your cold remedy herb. That's right, the echinacea you keep in the cupboard to ward off colds and flu may also help you clear up your complexion. It's actually a traditional herbalist's remedy that has been shown in some animal studies to help speed wound healing, which may be why it works for blemishes. What's more, it has bacteria-killing compounds, lessens inflammation, and even eases wound pain. Just place a few drops of tincture onto a soft pad or cotton ball and dab it right on pimples or soak a soft cloth with brewed echinacea tea and use as a daily wash.

Feel minty fresh. Mint is refreshment for your face: It may help remove some of the oil that clogs your pores and turns into unsightly blemishes. To make this herbal remedy, add the contents of two peppermint tea bags (or if available, 2 tablespoons of finely chopped fresh mint) to 2 tablespoons of plain unsweetened yogurt and 2 tablespoons of plain oatmeal (just whir some oats—not flavored

To pop or not?

Squeezing pimples or blackheads can increase inflammation, lead to infection, and cause skin damage, which can leave you with scarring and pitting. But if you can't stand the ugly whitehead for one minute longer, use the dermatologist-approved way for making it disappear. You'll need a needle, some rubbing alcohol, a cotton swab, and some hydrogen peroxide. Here's how to do it.

Clean the area. Take a needle and swab it with alcohol to sterilize it. Gently prick the

pimple. Use the swab to drain it. Clean it up with hydrogen peroxide, which is an antiseptic.

To remove a blackhead, you can find a tool called a blackhead extractor in the drugstore. Soften the area for 10 minutes with a hot-water compress (not so hot that you'll burn yourself). Then wash your hands well (keep scrubbing with soap and water until you finish reciting the alphabet) before using the extractor to reduce infection risk.

or instant—in your blender or food processor until finely powdered). Mix all the ingredients together and leave them on your face for 10 minutes, then wash off with plain water and dry.

Mash an aspirin. Aspirin contains salicylic acid, an old frontline remedy for acne. Aspirin helps reduce inflammation and dries up pimples. Mash an aspirin with a little water to form a paste and dab it on a blemish, or use a solution made from four adult aspirin dissolved in 2 tablespoons of water. (Make sure to use uncoated aspirin tablets.) You can also take an aspirin orally to help get the red out, but always check with your doctor before you start taking the drug regularly.

Consult the witch. Witch hazel, that is. Pour a little witch hazel onto a cotton ball to clean your face morning and night. Witch hazel is a natural astringent that helps to dry and shrink pimples.

Hit it with healthy acids. Any acidic fruit juice (lemon, lime, grapefruit) or vinegar can help flush pores. Dab onto acne with a cotton ball or swab.

Make a blackhead eradicator. To get rid of those tiny dark skin spots that look like specks of pepper, add 1 teaspoon of Epsom salts and 3 drops of iodine to ½ cup of water and bring to a boil. Let cool. Dip in a clean cotton pad and use it to clean your pores.

Fight oil with fat. But not just any fat—use the omega-3 fatty acids found in fish. One study found that people taking a multi-nutrient capsule containing fish oil had significantly less acne than they did before they started the remedy. Omega-3s are anti-inflammatory, and acne is all about inflammation. Fatty fish such as canned salmon, sardines, albacore tuna, and mackerel, and other foods such as flaxseed and walnuts are high in these healthy oils. Your acne RX: Two to three fish meals a week, or sprinkle a spoonful of freshly ground flaxseed on cereal or salads, and pop walnuts as a snack.

Relax and soothe with chamomile. The same tea you drink to reduce stress can lessen acne inflammation. Whir the contents of a chamomile tea bag in a blender or spice or coffee grinder, mix with just enough water to make a paste, and apply to inflamed skin. Or, brew up a strong

Weird & wacky

Early American settlers had some pretty strange notions when it came to eradicating acne. One involved the application of urine to the outbreaks. Another called for using the water that collected in old tree stumps to bathe pimpled skin. Needless to say, neither has been studied, and neither is worth trying.

chamomile tea with two tea bags to 1 cup boiled water. Cover and let steep for 15 minutes. Apply the cooled tea to your face with a cotton ball after cleansing.

 recipes for healing

Pimple-Relieving Compress

This gentle treatment will help send a pimple on its way.

> 4 teaspoons hot water
> 2 drops tea tree essential oil

1. Put the hot water in a bowl. Swirl the tea tree essential oil through the water, then soak a cotton ball or gauze pad in the solution.

2. Gently squeeze out excess liquid and apply the cotton ball or pad directly to the area of the pimple. Cover with plastic wrap and secure with a bandage or tape. Leave in place for at least an hour. Repeat twice a day.

Clarifying Herbal Hot Pack

This soothing treatment will open pores and kill bacteria.

> 4 green tea bags
> 1 tablespoon dried thyme
> 1 tablespoon dried oregano
> 1 quart water

1. Put tea bags, thyme, oregano, and water in a pot and bring to a boil.

2. Cover and steep for at least 60 minutes.

3. Reheat after an hour until it's almost too hot to touch, then saturate a clean cotton face towel until soaked through.

4. Carefully wring out the towel, and gently place on your face. Sit back and relax for 10 to 20 minutes. For best results, soak towel in the hot tea again whenever it cools off.

allergies

If you step outside and are immediately sneezing, sniffling, and rubbing your eyes, you're not allergic to the great outdoors—you're allergic to the pollen, dust, or mold floating in the air. All manner of harmless things, from your pet cat to peanuts, can make you react as if they were dangerous toxins. There's no cure for allergies, but you can reduce and treat your symptoms naturally with remedies you make yourself from stuff you already have in the house. Happy breathing!

first things first

There are lots of tricks for avoiding allergens. Here are several popular ones for the most common allergy triggers, including dust, mold, and pollen:

• Keep indoor humidity levels below 35 percent to prevent growth of mold and mites.

• Stay in the air-conditioning during pollen season.

• If you can, hire someone to mow the lawn.

• Breathe through your nose, not your mouth, to help filter out pollen.

• Immediately shower and wash your hair after coming inside.

• After spending time outdoors, immediately wash your clothes to prevent bringing pollen inside.

• Create an asthma-safe and allergy-free garden, using female plants (no pollen), pollen-free grass, and plants without strong perfume.

Pantry HEALERS

Apples

Black, green, and
  white tea

Chili peppers

Fish

Garlic

Greens

Honey

Horseradish

Lemon tea

Olives

Onions

Nuts

Red wine

Salt

Thyme

Wheat germ

If you've never had allergies before or if home remedies, over-the-counter antihistamines, or prescription medications aren't working, or if you're wheezing, it's time to make an appointment.

It may be time to call for emergency help if you have trouble breathing, experience swelling of your lips or throat, feel dizzy or light-headed, or have gastrointestinal symptoms. In severe form, those are the symptoms of anaphylactic shock, more common with food allergies than respiratory allergies.

the natural
DOCTOR'S R_x

Painful as it may be to your allergic child, get rid of her stuffed animals, and consider finding nonallergenic replacements. Also consider eliminating drapes, carpeting, decorative pillows, or other decorative accessories that attract dust and allergens.

• In spring and early summer, avoid exercising in the evening when you're more likely to breathe in pollen and pollutants.

• In late summer and fall, don't exercise in the morning when pollen counts are highest.

• Use a vacuum with a high-efficiency particulate air (HEPA) filter.

• If you have pets, don't let them in your bedroom, and wash them once a week.

• Choose washable throw rugs instead of wall-to-wall carpeting.

• Run a dehumidifier in your basement to remove moisture and prevent mold.

• Get a plastic, dust-proof cover for your mattress to thwart dust mites.

• Wash bed linens once a week in hot water or dry in a hot dryer to kill mites.

• Don't put plants in your bedroom.

• Use exhaust fans in the kitchen and bathroom to remove excess moisture and odors from the air.

• Get rid of unnecessary stuffed animals, drapes, carpeting, and pillows. All harbor dust and allergens.

kitchen cabinet cures

Have tea in bed. A nice hot cup of steaming lemon tea with honey in the morning will wake up your nasal cilia, the itty-bitty hairs in your nose that whisk pollen and dust out of your nasal passages. If you have allergies, those cilia are liable to be sluggish. A cup of tea will rouse the cilia to keep pollen and air particles at bay so you're not sneezing and coughing first thing in the morning. Add a little sage, fennel, or anise from your spice rack to help stimulate your nasal cilia even more.

In fact, have tea any old time. Black, green, and white teas are rich in flavonoids, plant chemicals that protect against inflammation.

Cue into quercetin. This plant chemical is also a flavonoid, a plant compound that's been found to protect us against everything from heart disease and cancer to cataracts, allergies, and asthma. In test tubes, it prevents immune cells from releasing histamine. You can take a supplement, but quercetin comes in some attractive food packages, including tea, red wine, apples, garlic, and onions.

Go Mediterranean. A study of children living in Crete, Greece, found far fewer allergies and less asthma among those who ate the healthy Greek diet—fish, loads of vegetables and fruit, olive oil, and nuts. Among the most protective foods in their diets were nuts. Of course, make sure your child doesn't have an allergy to nuts before adding these to her diet.

Sprinkle on the wheat germ. In one study, men and women with allergy symptoms who took 800 IU of vitamin E every day (in addition to taking their regular allergy meds) discovered they didn't need as much medication as similar sufferers who took a placebo, particularly for stuffiness. Vitamin E is a potent antioxidant that appears to calm the part of the immune system involved in allergies. You can certainly reach for the vitamin E in your kitchen vitamin drawer, but studies suggest being cautious about taking more than 400 IU, the amount found in the average multivitamin. Get the rest from food. Wheat germ is one of the best sources. Mix it into cereal, oatmeal, salads, meatloaf, or casseroles. To increase your vitamin E intake further, snack on almonds, hazelnuts, peanuts, and pistachios. Peanut butter also supplies vitamin E, as do fortified cereals.

Unstuff with horseradish. You know it makes your eyes water and your nose run, but there's also scientific evidence that this spicy root may act as a natural decongestant. Spread some jarred horseradish on whole-wheat crackers—it tastes better than you think!

Find some folate. This B vitamin is abundant in fortified whole-grain products, as well as in canned, dark green veggies like canned spinach, collard or mustard greens, and canned peas. A study of the diets of more than 8,000 American adults and children found that those who had the least folate in their diets were the most likely to have high levels of antibodies to pollen, dust mites, and animal dander, and to have wheezing problems, a symptom of asthma.

Weird & wacky

Actually, this remedy for hay fever may not be as wacky as it sounds—it's endorsed by many reputable healers, and it's a popular treatment in England. Honey that's produced locally—say, within 25 miles of your home—may contain pollen from the plants that trigger your allergies. If you eat a spoonful or so of this honey daily during the winter, it's just possible that it could act similarly to allergy shots and blunt your allergic reaction. We think it's a sweet remedy that can't hurt and just might help. (Note: Never give honey to babies under a year old.)

Eating hot peppers can help battle allergies by making nasal passages less sensitive.

Chow down on chili. The capsaicin in the chili pepper may calm the inner lining of the nasal passages (called the mucosa), making them less sensitive to irritants and less likely to become inflamed and secrete the protective fluids that stuff you up. And if you've ever eaten a hot pepper, you know it will help clear your nasal passages pronto.

Make a saline solution. Mixing ¼ teaspoon salt and ¼ teaspoon baking soda in 8 ounces of warm water. Place the saline solution in the neti pot, and, tipping your head to one side, pour the solution into one nostril. It will run into the other nostril and down the back of your throat. Drain by spitting out the remnants and blowing your nose.

This simple treatment will remove irritants and even some inflammatory cells from your nose. Use it at least once a day, and make sure to give yourself a rinse when you come in from the outdoors to wash pollens away.

Make a hay fever inhaler. Old-time herbalists believed that inhaling certain brews could ease allergy symptoms. They had a point: The herb in this brew contains thymol. Research shows that thymol reduces bronchial tract swelling and has anti-inflammatory and some antibacterial action. To make it, put ½ ounce dried thyme in a 1-pint canning jar and cover with boiling water. Close the jar tightly. Let steep and cool for 30 minutes. Remove the lid. Breathe in the vapors deeply several times. Keep the jar with you and inhale as needed during the day.

If you're allergic to what you eat

The most common food allergies are to the proteins in cow's milk, eggs, peanuts, wheat, soy, fish, shellfish, and tree nuts (like walnuts or almonds). If you break out in hives, have respiratory symptoms, or are likely to go into anaphylactic shock after eating the offending food, you need to be vigilant:

• Always ask about ingredients when you are eating away from home, such as in a restaurant or at someone else's house.

• Read food labels and know what you're looking for. Soy can be soy or it can be "natural flavorings." When in doubt, avoid the product until you contact the manufacturer.

• Always carry antihistamines or injectable epinephrine with you in case you eat something by accident. You should also wear an ID bracelet that describes your allergy.

arthritis

Almost everyone gets a "touch" of arthritis as they age. Usually it's osteoarthritis, a joint disease caused by the wear and tear of a life filled with tennis games, toting kids, and even that great fitness program you've stuck to all these years. Rheumatoid arthritis, on the other hand, is a painful, joint-disfiguring condition that occurs when your immune system mistakes normal tissue for something foreign and attacks it. It can occur at any age. Drugs—some powerful—will help, but some easy, soothing home remedies also carry the promise of a pain-free life.

first things first

There's more to treating arthritis than just alleviating pain when it occurs. Doctors increasingly are recommending that people with arthritis go on an anti-inflammatory diet. That means nixing foods that trigger inflammation. On the no-no list are the usual suspects: fast foods, junk foods, fried foods, and processed foods. Instead, adopt a healthy Mediterranean-style diet with plenty of fresh fruits and veggies, fish, olive oil, garlic, onions, and herbs. A Swedish study of patients with rheumatoid arthritis found that those who switched to the Mediterranean eating plan had less inflammation and regained some physical function as a result.

To start improving your diet right away, look to your pantry for nuts, dried fruits, canned fruits (in juice, not sugary syrups), canned fish, and whole grains such as barley, oats, tabbouleh, couscous, and brown rice.

Pantry HEALERS

Capsaicin

Cayenne

Chamomile

Cloves

Eucalyptus
    essential oil

Ginger tea

Green tea

Lavender

Rice

Rosemary

Thyme

Turmeric

Vanilla
    essential oil

Since you can't be sure what
kind of arthritis you have
or whether your symptoms
suggest another condition
entirely, see your doctor if
joint stiffness, swelling, redness, or pain persists more
than a few days—especially if
it becomes red, hot, swollen,
and very painful. You could
have gout (in which uric acid
crystals collect in the joint,
causing inflammation). You're
at risk for gout if you're overweight, if your diet is loaded
with red meat, or if you're a
heavy beer or spirits drinker.
Sometimes, infections are
responsible for joint pain.

If you've already been diagnosed with arthritis, call your
doctor if you notice a different
type of swelling in your joints.

kitchen cabinet cures

Fill your socks with rice. No, not while you have them on! Fill a cotton sock (there's a microwave involved, so you don't want a synthetic fiber that will melt) with any kind of uncooked rice you have in your cabinet and seal it. Put it in the microwave on high for 2 to 3 minutes. Remove carefully—it will be hot. When it cools down slightly but is still nice and warm, place it on a sore, stiff joint for pain relief. It should stay warm for about half an hour. You'll love how the rice shapes to your body and provides sooth-ing heat. If you have some lavender or other fragrant herb on hand, toss it in for a little relaxing aromatherapy, too. Reuse as often as you wish.

Sip some ginger tea. Numerous studies have found that ginger mimics nonsteroidal anti-inflammatories (NSAIDS), the front-line drugs for arthritis. It seems to work by curbing pain-causing chemicals that are part of the body's inflammatory response—and does it without the side effects of medication. Use powdered, raw, or lightly cooked fresh ginger liberally on food. Make tea by slicing three or four quarter-sized pieces of ginger into a couple of cups of boiling water. Simmer, covered, for 15 minutes and enjoy two or three times a day. You can also pick up ginger tea bags at the supermarket or health food store.

Make some spice rack rubs. Add a little cayenne, rose-mary, or thyme to ½ cup of olive or vegetable oil and use it as a soothing rub. All these herbs have pain-soothing properties.

Give joints the cold-hot treatment. You'll need two containers: Fill one with cold water and a tray of ice cubes, the other with hot water at a temperature you can tolerate to touch. Always start with cold, and immerse the hurting joint for a minute, then switch to the hot water and immerse for 30 seconds. After this, switch from cold to hot for about 15 minutes, immersing the affected joint in each for 30 sec-onds each time. Finish with cold water for a minute.

Wash the dishes. If your hands ache, this simple kitchen task is just what the doctor ordered. First, you're dipping your hands in hot water, which can help relax muscles and joints and relieve stiffness. Second, you're exercising your hands, which helps keep your hands and fingers mobile.

Turn on the kitchen radio. Study after study has found that listening to your favorite music can ease the ache, in part by distracting you and in part by raising levels of hormones that reduce your pain sensitivity. In one Cleveland Clinic Foundation study of people with back, neck, or joint pain, one group was given a play list of relaxing tunes, a second group chose their own sound track, and a third didn't get a musical prescription. The two music groups had lower rates of arthritis pain, depression, and disability than the non-music group, which experienced a 2 percent rise in pain. The study also indicated that the kind of music you listen to doesn't matter. Classical, country, or hip-hop—you just have to like it. The people who chose their own pain-relief tunes experienced a greater reduction in pain, depression, and disability than those who listened to generic relaxing music.

Sniff some pretty spices. Studies have found that pleasant aromas like lavender can alter the perception of pain. Japanese researchers think they know why: They found that lavender reduces levels of the stress hormone cortisol, which can make you feel relaxed and less likely to be aware of pain. But lavender isn't the only pleasant aroma that works. In one study, Korean researchers found that people with arthritis had less pain and were less depressed when exposed to the aromas of a variety of kitchen spices, including marjoram, rosemary, and peppermint. Make a pain-soothing blend to inhale by adding a teaspoon or so of one of these dried herbs to a quarter-cup of vegetable oil. Take a whiff frequently.

Make your own capsaicin cream. This old home remedy is now an over-the-counter treatment for arthritis and back pain. A substance extracted from spicy cayenne pepper, capsaicin reduces levels of a compound called substance P, which transmits pain signals to the brain. You can whip up some kitchen cabinet relief by mixing a few dashes of ground cayenne with 2 to 3 teaspoons of olive oil. Apply it with gauze to unbroken skin at the painful joints several times a day. The first few doses will cause a mild burning sensation, but you'll become desensitized after a week or so. Just keep it away from the mouth, eyes, and other mucous membranes, and avoid direct contact with the pepper's seeds—cayenne is highly irritating. Mild skin irritation is a common side effect of this treatment.

Pain-relieving perfume

There's no more convenient place to stash your favorite pain-relieving scent than on your skin. You can easily whip up a skin oil that will be there—right on your arm or wrist—when you really need it.

Take 15 drops of an essential oil known to relieve pain—lavender, chamomile, eucalyptus, or vanilla—and mix it with about 2 tablespoons of a neutral oil like almond, jojoba, coconut, or avocado. Dab on your skin. You can also use it as massage oil.

Don't use the same scented oil every day. You'll soon get used to the scent and will no longer respond to its pain-relieving ability.

An old cure for "rheuma-
tism" was to kill a rattlesnake
before it had a chance to
strike (always a good idea),
skin it, dry it, and then put
the remains in a jug of corn
whiskey. Then, drink the
whiskey. No surprise: There's
no science to support this
(and it's a little too dangerous
to recommend). But there
have been studies at Israel's
Shulov Institute for Science
looking at the possibility that
snake venom, with toxins
removed, could become a
potential remedy for arthritis. Venom contains certain
peptides—molecules containing amino acids—that can
turn off pain signals, which
is handy for a reptile that
needs to immobilize its prey.
Of course, there's a fine line
between momentary paraly-
sis and death, so we don't
want you trying this one
at home.

Apply a chamomile tea poultice. Along with calming your nerves, chamomile tea is an anti-inflammatory that may help ease arthritis pain. Brew a strong infusion using four chamomile tea bags in a cup or so of hot water. Steep, covered, for 20 minutes, then squeeze and remove tea bags. Soak a clean cloth in the liquid and apply. One caveat: If you're allergic to ragweed, asters, or chrysanthemums, you may be allergic to chamomile.

Go green. Sip four cups of green tea a day. In a recent study conducted at Case Western Reserve University, researchers gave mice the equivalent of four cups of green tea a day. Then they gave the mice a substance that would normally produce rheumatoid arthritis. The tea-drinking mice were far less likely to develop arthritis than the mice that drank water. Other research found that tea's polyphenols—antioxidant properties—were also anti-inflammatory and improved arthritis-related immune responses.

Stir in some turmeric. Researchers have discovered that turmeric—the yellow spice found in curries and ball-park mustard—contains a powerful compound called curcumin, which inhibits enzymes and proteins that promote inflammation. Several studies have found that turmeric specifically reduces pain and swelling in people with arthritis. In one study of people with knee osteoarthritis, those who ate just 2 grams a day (less than a teaspoon) had pain relief and increased mobility equal to those who took 800 milligrams of ibuprofen, an over-the-counter nonsteroidal anti-inflammatory. Sprinkle about ½ teaspoon on rice or in vegetables daily. Or keep some packets of ballpark mustard in your pocket—they're the perfect dose.

Clove up! Cloves contain an anti-inflammatory chemical called eugenol that interferes with a bodily process that's linked to the kind of immune response that triggers arthritis. In one animal study, eugenol prevented the release of COX-2, a protein that spurs inflammation. That's the same protein that COX-2 inhibitor drugs like celecoxib (Celebrex) target. In another, clove compounds inhibited the inflammation process involved in conditions like arthritis, asthma, and allergies, to name a few. Cloves also contain antioxidants, important in slowing the cartilage and bone damage caused by arthritis. Cloves are used liberally in Indian cuisine and spice up everything from stew to meat loaf and even quick breads. Aim for ½ to 1 teaspoon a day.

Stick to low-allergenic foods. There's some evidence that food allergies may play a part in autoimmune illnesses like rheumatoid arthritis. At the University of Oslo in Norway, researchers found that people with the autoimmune disease had higher levels of antibodies to cow's milk, eggs, codfish, and pork than people who didn't have the disease. In one study, people with rheumatoid arthritis who followed a diet that eliminated common allergens like grains (especially gluten-containing wheat products), nuts, milk, and eggs for 10 to 18 days had significant symptomatic improvement. When they started eating these foods again, they felt worse. Other studies have found that corn, wheat, oranges, oats, rye, eggs, beef, and coffee may also be problem foods. Interestingly, many of these foods help produce arachidonic acid, a body chemical that's linked to inflammation.

 recipes for healing

Gingery Poultice

Applying crushed ginger to a painful joint can deplete the body's stores of substance P, a brain chemical that carries pain messages to your central nervous system. One study of 56 people found that ginger eased symptoms in 55 percent of people with osteoarthritis and 74 percent of those with rheumatoid arthritis.

   3-inch piece of fresh ginger
   Olive oil

1. Peel and finely mince the ginger.

2. Mix it with just enough olive oil to form a paste.

3. Apply to the painful joint. Depending on where the pain is, you may need to wrap the ginger in place with a gauze or Ace bandage. Leave in place for 10 to 15 minutes. Don't wrap too tightly. For extra relief, gently warm the ginger before applying.

Minty Pain Relief Oil

Hard to believe that the most ubiquitous flavor in the world—it's in your toothpaste!—can also kill pain. In one study, peppermint oil rubbed on the forehead and temples of chronic headache sufferers eased their pain. Mint is also a traditional ingredient of salves and oils for soothing aching muscles.

> 2 cups, more or less, fresh mint leaves
> Olive oil
> 1 tablespoon vodka or rubbing alcohol
> Few drops tincture of benzoin

1. Loosely fill a small clean jar with fresh mint leaves.
2. Cover with olive oil to fill the jar.
3. Add the vodka or rubbing alcohol. Allow it to sit on a sunny window and steep for at least 2 weeks. Then strain it and transfer it to a clean jar or bottle. Add the tincture of benzoin (available at drugstores and health food stores) to preserve the oil. Store it in a cool dark place. Rub onto aching joints as needed.

Spicy Massage Oil

This rub is packed with herbs that relieve pain and inflammation. Use it twice a day, every day, for a week or until pain abates.

> 1 tablespoon dried rosemary leaves
> 3 teaspoons celery seeds
> 1 teaspoon crushed cayenne or other red pepper
> 8 ounces olive, almond, or jojoba oil

1. Whir the rosemary, celery seeds, and red pepper until pulverized in a clean coffee or spice grinder.
2. Spoon into a glass jar with a tight-fitting lid and add the oil.
3. Shake vigorously, then cover and leave for 10 days, shaking periodically.
4. Strain through a paper coffee filter into a sterilized glass bottle and keep in a cool, dark place for up to 6 months, longer if you refrigerate it.
5. To use: Rub 1 to 2 drops onto the skin to test for any adverse reaction. If there is no reaction, gently massage a little of the oil onto the aching joint twice a day.

athlete's foot

That itching, burning sensation in your sneakers means that a fungus called tinea pedis is taking up residence between your toes. (Yes, go ahead and say, "Ewww!") Athlete's foot also causes blisters, scaling, oozing, and crusting and, if left untreated, can spread to your heels, palms, and between your fingers. Fortunately, nature has provided a plethora of antifungals and soothing remedies that you probably already store right in your kitchen.

first things first

A few basics can help protect feet from the infernal itch. These are tops on our list if your feet are prone to athlete's foot:

• Regularly wash your feet with soap and water or use a basin of water with about an ounce of vinegar added. Pay special attention to the space between your toes where tinea fungus love to settle.

• What's good for a baby's bottom is good for your tootsies, too. After washing and drying feet well, sprinkle on some talcum, cornstarch, or antifungal powder.

• Be selective about footwear. You may love the latest celebrity-endorsed sports shoe, but if it's all leather, it could turn into a steamy condo for fungus.

• When your feet sweat, you want socks that will wick the moisture away, and cotton socks—well, they just stay wet. Wear sports socks specially designed to keep your feet dry.

Pantry HEALERS

Aloe

Baking soda

Cloves

Mustard powder

Onion juice

Oregano

Tea tree oil

Thyme

Vinegar

Yogurt

If you have diabetes and a case of athlete's foot, make an appointment. The disease can cause circulation problems and nerve damage that make any wound or infection more serious.

Call your physician if you notice your feet are warm to the touch, swollen, or have red streaks, all symptomatic of infection. Ditto if a fever or pus or other discharge accompanies the condition. Finally, consult your doctor if you've tried lots of remedies and the condition doesn't go away. Stronger antifungal medication may be your only solution.

• If your feet sweat a lot, change your socks a couple of times a day and alternate pairs of shoes to allow them time to dry out. You may need to do this more frequently with shoes and socks you use during exercise.

• Never go barefoot in public places! Wear sandals or water shoes, especially in gym showers or at the pool.

• But go barefoot at home. Going shoeless around the house will allow your feet to dry and "breathe," which will discourage fungal growth.

kitchen cabinet cures

Let baking soda quench the burning itch. Add enough water to 1 tablespoon of baking powder to make a paste. Rub it on the parts of your foot that itch. It will provide quick relief. Let the paste sit for 5 to 10 minutes, then rinse thoroughly and dry your feet completely. Dust your piggies with talc or cornstarch afterward.

Try powdered mustard. Put a tablespoon or so of mustard powder from your spice rack into a warm footbath and give your feet a good, long soak. Mustard has antifungal properties.

Dunk those dogs in yogurt. The live acidophilus bacteria in yogurt send in friendly microorganisms to vanquish the unfriendly fungus that's causing the burning, itching, and flaking between your toes. Dab a little plain yogurt on the affected areas, let it dry, then rinse off and dry thoroughly.

Give your feet and your socks the vinegar treatment. Soak a cotton ball in vinegar and dab affected areas several times a day. Likewise, kill fungus in your socks by soaking them in vinegar for a half an hour.

Fight odor with odor. An old home remedy that seems to have some merit is using fresh onion juice to treat athlete's foot. One reason it may work: Onions have antimicrobial properties, meaning they're the natural enemy of bacteria and fungi. To use, whir a roughly chopped onion in a food processor with enough water to make a paste. Place your feet in a basin and slather on the smelly slurry. Let it sit for 30 minutes or so before rinsing off and thoroughly drying your feet.

Try tea tree oil. If you don't have tea tree oil in your medicine cabinet, you should. It's an essential home remedy item for scores of problems. This potent antiseptic has been used for all kinds of skin conditions for more than a century. One study found that tea tree oil was as effective as an over-the-counter remedy for athlete's foot for relieving burning, itching, inflammation, and scaling. Add a few drops to a tablespoon of witch hazel and apply to the affected area with a cotton swab three times a day. It can cause dermatitis (skin inflammation) in some people, so use sparingly the first time and don't use further if a rash develops.

Give your feet some thyme. Mix up a cup of strong thyme tea (2 tablespoons of dried thyme to 8 ounces of boiling water, covered and steeped for 10 minutes). Strain it, and when it cools, soak a cotton cloth in the tea and wipe your feet, particularly the reddened areas and between your toes. Dry thoroughly with a clean cloth. Thyme has antifungal properties. You can also try the same brew substituting cloves or oregano, two other powerhouse antifungal agents in your spice rack. (For a one-two punch at the visiting fungi, dab tea tree oil diluted in a little witch hazel on afterward.)

|||||||||||||||||||||||||||||||||||||||||||||

Check your pet

If you've tried it all, and you *still* have athlete's foot, consider your pet. In one study of 211 dogs, researchers found 89 fungal strains on them that can infect humans. In fact, 11 dog owners who had athlete's foot or jock itch (infection of the groin area by the same group of fungi that cause athlete's foot) were infected with a fungus strain also carried by their pets. If you think your pet might be causing your fungal troubles, ask your veterinarian to check your canine or kitty.

 recipe for healing

Aloe Ointment

Aloe-based remedies bought at the drugstore are expensive, but are made from the same gel you get for free from the aloe plant on your windowsill.

> 1 aloe stalk
> ½ teaspoon tea tree oil
> 10 drops lavender oil

1. Slit the aloe stalk and use a teaspoon to scoop off all the gel.
2. Blend in the tea tree and lavender oils.
3. Rub the salve into the affected areas. The aloe helps heal raw, cracked skin, and the two oils fight fungi. Use as often as necessary.

back pain

Pantry HEALERS

Canned fish

Cherries

Dark chocolate

Flaxseed

Fruits and vegetables

Nuts

Olive oil

Tea

Vanilla

Vitamin D

Walnuts

If you've never had back pain, you belong to a very small club. As many as 8 out of 10 people have had an aching back at some time in their lives. Often, the pain is just the result of an injury—a fall on the ice, lifting a too-heavy load, twisting in a way the body was not designed to twist. A little ice, a little heat, and a few days of painkillers and the problem is over. But for too many of us, back pain is an ongoing dilemma. There are many natural ways to ease the hurt when it happens and keep it from happening in the first place. Here are many of a kitchen-cabinet nature.

first things first

Home remedies have their place in dealing with back pain, but when it really hurts, start with these steps:

• Apply a heating pad for 20 to 30 minutes at a time. Or use the hot rice-sock remedy detailed in the Arthritis section.

• Use an over-the-counter pain medication, such as acet-aminophen, ibuprofen, naproxen, or ketoprofen.

• To take pressure and weight off your back, lie on your back with pillows under your knees and your hips and knees bent. You can also rest your feet on a chair from that position.

• Don't rest longer than one or two days. Bed rest can weaken your muscles even further. Try to walk around as much as possible.

- To reduce any curve in your spine, sleep on your side with your knees bent. You can also put a pillow between your knees. If you're a back sleeper, make sure you have a pillow under your knees and your lower back.

- Avoid sleeping on your stomach unless you have a pillow under your hips.

kitchen cabinet cures

Get your daily D. One of the little-known contributors to back pain is lack of vitamin D, the "sunshine" vitamin. In one study, more than 80 percent of people between the ages of 15 and 52 who had chronic low back pain were deficient in this vitamin, which is necessary for maintaining normal levels of calcium in the blood. When they supplemented their diets with vitamin D, their back pain improved. And in the small number of people with normal vitamin D levels, 69 percent also experienced less pain when they took extra vitamin D.

The best way to get vitamin D is to spend 15 minutes a day three times a week in the sun, although for people in

When to Call THE DOCTOR

If you try traditional methods, plus one or more kitchen cabinet cures, and still have pain after two to three weeks, check in with your doc. Do so as well if you have any numbness or pain that travels down your leg or if pain is so intense you can't move. Likewise, give the doc a call if an injury triggered the pain or if you have other symptoms such as fever, nausea, vomiting, abdominal distress, weakness, or sweating.

Eat away back pain

Certain foods can quench the inflammation that contributes to all kinds of pain. Your back pain diet should include:

- Olive oil

- Canned salmon, sardines packed in water or olive oil, mackerel, albacore tuna, flaxseed, walnuts

- Cherries. One study showed that drinking 12 ounces of tart cherry juice twice a day for eight days, reduced muscle pain and strain. Canned tart cherries, packed in their own juice, would also be helpful.

- Vegetable protein (such as soy)

- Vegetables and fruits of every hue—canned or frozen are fine, as long as they're not packed with heavy syrup or salt

- Nuts

- Tea

- Dark chocolate in moderation (1 ounce a day)

Then, there are the foods NOT to eat. These foods can increase inflammation inside the body, fanning the pain:

- Vegetable oils such as corn, safflower, sunflower, cottonseed, and mixed vegetable oils

- Margarine and vegetable shortening

- Processed foods

- Products containing high-fructose corn syrup

- Saturated fats, including meat, butter, and full-fat dairy products

- Foods made with trans fats

northern climes the sun may not be strong enough to activate the vitamin D raw material that's stored in the skin. And getting that much sun can be nearly impossible during winter months. Some nutrition experts suggest taking 1,000 IU of vitamin D_3 every day.

Hit the vanilla. Dab a few drops of vanilla onto a handkerchief and sniff it to make the pain go away. It will help relieve your stress, which can exacerbate pain of any kind. A study done at the Columbia University Medical Center found that people who smelled vanilla while doing stress tests had more stable heart rates and lower blood pressure—markers of relaxation—than those who took the same tests without any exposure to scent. If you're tense, studies have found, you can be more pain-sensitive.

Listen to the kitchen radio. A study done at the Cleveland Clinic Foundation found that people with back and other kinds of aches who listened to music they enjoyed for an hour a day experienced a 25 percent decrease in their pain. Researchers aren't sure if it's relaxation or distraction that does the trick, but if you're in pain, music can be, well, music to your ears.

Weird & wacky

We just love this old North Carolinian folk remedy for a bad back: Lie down (presumably outside) and when you hear the call of a whip-poor-will, roll over three times. This remedy may have been inspired by one that hails from Sussex, England. There, folkloric advice calls for the back pain sufferer to roll on the ground at the sound of spring's first cuckoo. We suspect the rolling had something to do with stretching out sore back muscles—and birdsong is one of the best soul lifters around.

recipes for healing

Classic Mustard Plaster

You may remember this one from your childhood. It worked well when you had chest congestion, and it works equally well on back pain.

> 2 or more tablespoons white or brown mustard seeds, ground in coffee grinder
> (or 2 tablespoons powdered mustard, such as Coleman's)
> 3 tablespoons flour
> 1 egg white
> 1–4 tablespoons warm water

1. Stir the mustard and flour together in a small bowl.
2. Blend in the egg white and add enough water to form a thick paste.
3. Spread the mustard plaster on a cloth or paper towel.
4. Have someone place the cloth or towel on your back, mustard side on the skin, and leave on for about 20 minutes. Mustard seeds act like a counter-irritant to help reduce pain, much like over-the-counter capsaicin creams.

Camphor Oil Rub for Back Pain

You don't have to shell out dough for an over-the-counter cream for back pain. Instead, try this effective, easy-to-make rub.

> 1 tablespoon finely minced fresh ginger (or 1 tablespoon powdered ginger)
> 1 tablespoon dried rosemary
> ¼ cup olive oil
> 5 drops peppermint oil (optional)
> 2 drops camphor or wintergreen essential oil (optional)

1. Whir the ginger and rosemary in a clean coffee grinder till very fine and blended.
2. Mix the olive oil and the peppermint and camphor oils together in a small bowl.
3. Blend in the rosemary-ginger mixture.
4. Have someone rub the fragrant mixture into the painful area of your back and cover with a piece of flannel or an old T-shirt. Then put a heating pad over the cloth for 15–20 minutes and rest while the rubs soak in. You can double the recipe for larger areas. Wash it off during a soak in the tub, if you like.

body odor

When the answer to the question, "What's that terrible smell?" is "Yikes! It's me!" it's time to take some action. Though a dousing of perfume might replace one smell with a more pleasant one, it's probably better to attack the problem at a more fundamental level. And you can do it with ease, naturally.

first things first

These may seem painfully obvious, but just in case, here's a basic checklist to perform before you try more involved remedies:

• Wash daily. Use an antibacterial soap to stifle the bugs that make you smell in the first place.

• Dry thoroughly, especially your feet. Bacteria love damp spaces, such as the gaps between your toes, so give various parts of your body a blast from your hair dryer for about 30 seconds after bathing to make sure you are really dry.

• Use antiperspirant if you tend to sweat. These products block pores that produce sweat under the arms.

• But if you rarely sweat, use deodorant. It makes your skin acidic, which discourages bacterial growth. It usually contains perfume to mask odor. And yes, you can use it on other parts of your body that generate odor.

• Wear natural fibers. Cotton, wool, and silk allow your skin to breathe. If you exercise (and/or sweat) a lot, choose clothing designed to wick moisture away from the body.

Pantry HEALERS

Baking soda

Chamomile

Hydrogen peroxide

Lavender

Lemon

Parsley

Peppermint

Rosemary

Sage

Rubbing alcohol

Vinegar

Witch hazel

kitchen cabinet cures

Tone down the garlic and onions. Though we often recommend these two for their power to prevent infections, take them off the pantry shopping list if you have body-odor issues. They're not only the cause of bad breath, but in some folks, their scent can literally ooze out of their pores. Cumin is another body odor culprit. You don't have to eliminate them from your diet—they're good for you. But if you're going to be in close quarters, take a temporary pass.

Drink some chamomile tea. Body odor is often caused when perspiration—which is odorless—meets bacteria on the skin. Exercise is the healthy reason for sweat. Stress, on the other hand, can cause your sweat glands to get busy as well. When you're feeling nervous, overwhelmed, and anxious, brew a cup of this chamomile tea, which will calm you down immediately. And no one will ever see—or smell—you sweat.

Have a baking soda bath. It removes odors in your fridge and works on you, too. Baking soda is also mildly antiseptic. Alternatively, use it as a dusting powder like you would use talcum.

Swab on sage. This herb, which you probably associate with poultry seasoning, has antibacterial and antiperspiration properties. Add a teaspoon or two of dried sage to a cup of boiling water, allow it to cool, and apply with a cloth to sweat-prone areas, avoiding the face and genitals. You can also drink a cup or two a day to cool you off, though pregnant women should abstain.

Slice a lemon. Like over-the-counter deodorants, acidic fruits can change the pH of your skin, making it a hostile environment for the bacteria that cause odor. Slice a lemon in half and rub under your armpits and on the soles of your feet.

Have a witch hazel splash. Apply this astringent (drying), deodorizing liquid directly to your skin or apply with a cotton pad.

Hit on the germs. Use rubbing alcohol, vinegar, or hydrogen peroxide on underarms to discourage bacteria.

When to Call THE DOCTOR

Nearly all cases of body odor are harmless and the causes obvious. But in rare cases, body odors are an indication of a more serious condition. Call your doctor if:

• You suddenly develop a strong, unusual body odor. This is characteristic of kidney failure or a condition called diabetic ketoacidosis, in which you have too little insulin in your body to use glucose for energy.

• You smell like fish. You may have an uncommon genetic condition called trimethylaminuria, or fish odor syndrome, in which your body can't break down a nitrogen-containing compound in some foods.

• You smell like maple syrup. This is a symptom of—and we're not making this up—maple syrup urine disease, a genetic metabolic disorder in which your body can't metabolize certain amino acids. It's managed with a special diet, but if not diagnosed in time, can cause brain damage.

• You have unusual body odor and a rash. A bacterial infection called erythrasma is associated with a strong odor and brownish-red, scaly patches under the arms, in the groin area, or between the toes. It's treated with a topical antibiotic.

Weird & wacky

We wouldn't do this ourselves, but an old, traditional body-odor treatment was to add 2 or 3 cups of tomato juice to bathwater and soak in the solution for 15 minutes. The effectiveness of this harmless treatment has never been verified—but since it's also used for bathing dogs who've gotten "skunked," there must be something to it.

Make your own herbal bath solution. All you need is a piece of cheesecloth or a stocking, which you can fill with fragrant herbs of your choice, including lavender, sage, parsley, peppermint, or rosemary. Tie securely and toss into the tub. You can also rub the pouch over the areas where odor is problematic.

Pass on the hot stuff. Some foods, like chili peppers, can cause you to break out in a sweat. If smelly sweat is a problem for you, stay away from any food that increases it.

Chew on some parsley. This kitchen herb is 70 percent chlorophyll, which is known to clean up bad odors. It's also antibacterial. Nibble on a few sprigs after you've indulged in something especially odiferous.

 recipe for healing

Herbal Bath Deodorant

This lovely and fragrant bath will not only freshen you, but also will kill the bacteria that cause odor.

> 1 tablespoon dried rosemary
> 1 tablespoon dried sage
> 1 tablespoon dried peppermint
> 1 tablespoon dried lavender, if available

1. Whir the rosemary, sage, peppermint, and lavender in a clean coffee grinder.
2. Place them in a doubled piece of cheesecloth. Gather up the corners of the cheesecloth and tie securely.
3. Toss the bundle into a hot bath to scent the water. Rub the herbal pouch all over the skin, paying particular attention to areas where odor is a problem.

boils

It looks like a pimple on steroids, but a boil is a different kind of skin infection—usually caused by a specific bacteria called *Staphylococcus aureus*. They can be as small as a pea and as large as a golf ball and are most common on the face, neck, armpit, shoulders, and bottom, generally "boiling" up from a hair follicle or oil gland. They can be quite painful. But with a few home remedies, they can also be treated effectively.

first things first

When a boil boils up, start your home treatment simply:

• Dip a soft cloth into warm water and press against the boil for 20 minutes at least three or four times a day to encourage it to drain. Unless it drains, it can't heal. The heat also increases the amount of blood around the boil, sending more infection-fighting white blood cells to the site to fight it.

• Wash your hands frequently. Because boils are usually caused by a staph germ, you don't want to spread the infection to other parts of your body or other people in your life. Wash hands thoroughly with hot water and soap after touching the boil.

• Don't squeeze or pierce the boil. This can spread the infection.

• Take over-the-counter painkillers. Unlike most skin eruptions, boils can really hurt until they rupture, but a low dose of ibuprofen or acetaminophen can ease the pain.

Pantry HEALERS

Black tea
Chamomile
Epsom salts
Lavender
Oregano
Tea tree oil
Thyme
Turmeric

If a boil lasts longer than two weeks, feels warm, has red streaks stretching out from it, or is on the spine or the middle of the face, you may have a more serious infection that requires medical help. Likewise, if a boil is unusually deep or large, or there's more than one in the same area, you might need to have it lanced by a doctor.

Weird & wacky

This old English remedy, gets our vote for strangest of them all. Apply a poultice to the boil. When you remove the poultice, place it in a corpse-containing coffin. Theory was, the boils would leave you and pass on to the dead person, where they could do no harm.

kitchen cabinet cures

Add some natural antiseptics. Go plain water one better. Prepare a cup of thyme tea (1 teaspoon of dried thyme to 1 cup of boiling water) and use as a compress, particularly after the boil has ruptured. Thyme contains a natural antiseptic called thymol. Or try chamomile tea; it's anti-inflammatory and can ease redness and pain. Lavender and oregano also have antibacterial properties.

Try black tea. A plain warm tea bag can act as a compress, too—it contains tannins, which also have antibacterial properties.

Treat with tea tree oil. Studies have found that this oil from an Australian tree is highly effective against staph infections, even those that are antibiotic-resistant. Just dab a little on the boil several times a day.

Make a turmeric paste. An old Ayurvedic remedy from India involves making a paste of 4 to 5 tablespoons of the spice with water and applying it to the boil. Studies have found that turmeric is effective against staph and other common bacteria.

Soak with Epsom salts. Much as the salt you eat draws fluids into your bloodstream, a soaking solution of Epsom salts can draw fluid out of the skin, shrinking the underlying tissues and reducing inflammation. That's why Epsom salts are such a popular folk remedy for skin troubles, ranging from insect bites to poison ivy to boils.

 recipe for healing

Germ-Killing Poultice

¼ cup hot water
5 drops tea tree essential oil
5 drops lavender essential oil

1. Put the hot water in a bowl. Swirl the essential oils through the water, then soak a gauze pad in the solution.

2. Gently squeeze out excess fluid and apply it directly to the boil. Cover with plastic wrap and secure with a bandage or tape. Leave in place for at least an hour. Repeat twice a day.

bruises

You smacked into something—or something smacked into you—and you'll soon have an ugly purple splotch to mark the spot. If you race to the kitchen cabinet for some help, you just might be able to prevent the Technicolor display, or at least shorten the time it takes your bruise to fade from black. The key to bruise control is to take action quickly.

Pantry HEALERS

Arnica
Arrowroot
Castor oil
Lavender oil
Oregano
Sugar
Vinegar
Witch hazel

first things first

Kitchen cabinet cures really *are* effective for bruises. But always start with this approach: Press a cold, wet compress made of paper towels, napkins, handkerchiefs, or even tissues onto the bruise right away. Or wrap ice in a towel and firmly apply to the bruise (a bag of frozen veggies works in a pinch). This helps stop the bleeding under the skin and can lessen swelling.

kitchen cabinet cures

Add arnica to your kitchen cabinet. *Arnica montana* is an alpine flower with a long history of healing bruises and other wounds. Though you probably don't stock the stuff (or even know what it is), you should—especially if you have an active family. It's harmless, inexpensive, and when it works, it works really well. Buy arnica in homeopathic pill form at pharmacies and health-food stores. It comes in little vials that contain tiny sugar pills infused with minute doses of the herb. In 2006, plastic surgeons from a practice in Connecticut studied its effects on

We admit that this ancient Chinese treatment is probably more fun to read about than to use. And we can't vouch for its effectiveness. But it's harmless and may be worth a try—at the very least, it will amuse a bruised child and take his mind off his boo-boo. You need two things: a U.S. silver coin (dimes, quarters, and half dollars minted before 1964 are mostly silver) and a peeled, freshly hard-boiled egg. Slip the coin vertically all the way into the egg until its top edge is even with the top of the egg. Place the warm (not hot) egg on the bruise and leave it there for 30 minutes. This is said to immediately erase the discoloration.

29 people who'd just undergone face-lifts. They concluded that those who took arnica had smaller bruises than those who didn't. Key to success: Take it immediately after you've banged into something; the longer you wait, the less effective arnica is. Others swear by arnica cream. Spread it quickly on a bruise, as long as there aren't any cuts or scrapes on the site.

Lift the bruise with sweetness. This only works if you're close to the sugar bowl when you get bruised. Wet your fingers, dip them in sugar, and give the entire bruise a brisk, firm massage with your sugary fingers. This may help seal the capillaries that are bleeding under the skin and could prevent the bruise from forming.

Got some arrowroot? Many cooks keep this powder in the spice rack to thicken sauces. If you have some handy, take a tablespoon or two, depending on how large the bruised area is, add just enough water to make a paste, and slather it on the spot. When it dries, you may find that the bruise has disappeared.

Try vinegar. This remedy is as old as the hills, and like many folk remedies, no scientific studies exist to explain exactly how the sour liquid helps heal bruises. Simply mix equal parts of apple cider vinegar and warm water, soak a paper towel or cloth in the solution, and press it gently on the bruise. It's possible that the vinegar and warm water compress increases blood flow near the skin's surface. That could help dissipate the blood that has pooled in the area. Witch hazel will also do the trick.

Erase that black eye with castor oil. A shiner is embarrassing to explain, so short of making like a pirate and wearing an eye patch (which is even more embarrassing) try this: Gently massage castor oil on the discolored

Busting the pineapple myth

Think that eating lots of pineapple can help fade a bruise? Think again. It's true that bromelain, a natural substance found in pineapples, helps fade bruises because it has anticlotting and anti-inflammatory effects. Trouble is, you only find bromelain in pineapple stems, not in the yummy fruit. If you're planning surgery and want to minimize bruising, talk to your doctor about taking bromelain supplements.

skin. Be sure to keep the oil out of your eye. This is a tried and true folk remedy that's said to ease the pain, bring down the swelling, and lessen the unsightly color.

Rub in this simple massage oil. Mix 5 drops of lavender essential oil with 1 teaspoon vegetable oil, and massage into the bruise. The pressure of the massage will help the pooled blood reabsorb, and the scent of lavender will relax and calm you. Perfect for soothing your jangled nerves after a minor accident.

When to Call THE DOCTOR

Schedule a checkup if you're prone to large or painful bruises that appear for no apparent reason. Same goes if you begin bruising easily and start having nosebleeds or bloody gums.

 recipes for healing

Pizza Spice Poultice

This simple tea poultice can reduce the swelling and the pain of a bruise.

I heaping tablespoon dried oregano
I cup boiled water

1. Steep the oregano in the hot water for 10 minutes. Strain. Reserve the oregano and the liquid.

2. Wrap the damp oregano in a piece of cheesecloth roughly the size of the bruise to make a poultice.

3. Place the poultice on the bruise and leave it on for about 15 minutes. When the cheesecloth dries, re-wet it with the oregano water, and reapply.

Fragrant Oil Compress

This simple formula can ease an achy bruise, and it's a cinch to make. You can use all, one, or none of the essential oils, depending on what you have handy.

¼ cup water
¼ cup witch hazel or apple cider vinegar
5 drops lavender essential oil
5 drops rosemary essential oil
5 drops peppermint essential oil

1. In a bowl, mix together the water, witch hazel (or vinegar), and the essential oils. Soak a cloth in the liquid, wring it out until nearly dry, and then place over the injured area.

2. Cover with plastic wrap so the skin absorbs the essential oils, and cover the whole thing with a towel. Apply the compress for 30 minutes, and repeat up to three times daily.

canker sores

Pantry HEALERS

Aloe

Baking soda

Hydrogen peroxide

Licorice tea

Milk of magnesia

Sage

Tea

Tea tree oil

You've probably never called these mouth irritations by their real name, which is aphthous ulcers. But you've certainly had at least one or two of them in your lifetime. Stress, abrasions, and allergies are just a few causes for the sores, which, though annoying, are rarely cause for alarm. These kitchen cabinet cures should be able to shave at least a few days off their normal healing time, which is usually about a week.

first things first

Whether you have just one or a few canker sores, you'll want to apply some common-sense solutions in addition to the remedies below:

• Forego spicy or very acidic foods.

• Pass on crunchy or chewy foods.

• Rinse your mouth with salt water a few times a day.

• After brushing, rinse your mouth with an antibacterial mouthwash.

kitchen cabinet cures

Try aloe. Instead of buying an over-the-counter preparation in the drugstore to coat that painful canker sore, make your instant, natural cure. All you need is a cotton swab and an aloe vera leaf. Dry the sore area with a cotton swab, then slice into the leaf and scrape off a bit of gel with a clean spoon. Dab directly on the sore. Repeat as often as necessary.

Reach for baking soda. Rinse your mouth with a solution of 1 teaspoon baking soda in ½ cup of warm water. The baking soda helps kill the bacteria, which will ease the pain.

Use milk of magnesia. Sip a small amount and use it as a mouth rinse, making sure to rinse the canker sore itself. You can also dab milk of magnesia directly on the canker sore with a cotton swab three or four times a day.

Or, add this to the milk of magnesia. A variation on the milk of magnesia remedy above is to mix a teaspoon of it with a teaspoon of Benedryl liquid allergy medicine. Swish this blend around in your mouth.

Do the tea bag trick. Apply a damp tea bag to the sore for 5 minutes. Tea is alkaline, so it neutralizes acids. It also contains compounds that may help relieve pain.

Make like a sage. The culinary herb sage kills bacteria and viruses and contains compounds that reduce inflammation. Steep 2 teaspoons dried sage in a cup of boiling water, covered. Let cool, and use as a mouth rinse two or three times a day, making sure to swish the tea in the area of the mouth with the canker sore.

Climb the tea tree. Using a cotton swab, dab a single drop of tea tree oil, an antiseptic, directly on the sore.

When to Call THE DOCTOR

If you get more than your fair share of canker sores, let your doctor know so that he or she can rule out any medical problems. And make an appointment if your canker sores are so painful that you can't drink—you could become dehydrated, which is dangerous.

the natural DOCTOR'S Rx

Tasty licorice tea, which you can find in tea bags at health food stores, is an excellent way to treat and eliminate canker sores. Use one tea bag per cup of boiled water and steep, covered for 10 minutes, then drink.

recipe for healing

Disinfecting Mouth Rinse

Hydrogen peroxide is a strong disinfectant. That's a plus, since a canker sore is an open wound that's vulnerable to infection, which increases the pain. And since baking soda is alkaline, it provides extra relief by neutralizing acids.

¼ cup hydrogen peroxide
¼ cup water
1 teaspoon baking soda
1 teaspoon salt

1. Blend the peroxide and water in a glass.

2. Add the baking soda and salt and stir to dissolve thoroughly.

3. To use, swish the solution around in your mouth and spit it out.

carpal tunnel syndrome

Many people believe that carpal tunnel syndrome (CTS) is a condition of modern times, a result of countless hours spent typing on a computer keyboard. While research shows this isn't true, what's certain is that some old-fashioned kitchen remedies can help ease this increasingly common and painful wrist and hand problem.

first things first

Let's debunk the "computers are the primary cause of CTS" issue. A Mayo Clinic study found that people who use computers all day weren't at increased risk for developing this painful wrist or hand problem. More recently, a Danish study also concluded that there isn't enough evidence to blame computer work for CTS.

So who is at risk? According to a 2009 study, the likeliest victims of CTS are people who work in the meat or fish processing industries, foresters who work with chain saws, or workers on assembly lines producing electronic products. So while some office workers who spend lots of time on computers do get the condition, so do many other people who work far away from computers.

While home remedies and kitchen cabinet cures like the ones below can assist in fast and effective healing, you should also use these common-sense tactics:

• As with any inflammation-caused pain, heat and cold are your allies in relief. Apply an ice pack wrapped in a thin towel for 10 minutes to ease inflammation. You can repeat every hour. Once you are past the inflammation stage, use

Pantry HEALERS

Bromelain supplements

Canned fish (salmon, sardines, herring, mackerel)

Capsaicin cream

Caviar

Cayenne pepper

Flaxseed

heat to relax muscles. A warm bath before bed is a good approach.

• Stop doing the things that caused the damage to your wrists! If the repetitive task is job related, that might be hard. But at minimum, arrange at least a few days to let healing occur.

• If you have to keep doing the task after healing, alter your technique. Can you change how you grip the tool? The way you position your hands? Having more than one approach to a task can help prevent CTS.

• To ease the pain, stabilize the wrist with a splint. Wear as often as possible, but especially at night when you're apt to sleep in positions that can aggravate the inflammation (like with your hand under your pillow).

kitchen cabinet cures

Go salmon fishing. There are no studies as to whether eating fatty fish, such as canned salmon, sardines, herring, or mackerel can ease carpal tunnel syndrome. But since eating fatty fish is proven to have strong anti-inflammatory effects, it's a safe and healthy move to have two or three servings a week.

Scarf up some caviar. No, not the expensive stuff that will set you back a month's pay. Scientists recently discovered that salmon and lumpfish caviars are the food world's number one dietary source of inflammation-fighting omega-3 fatty acids. You can find these tasty, inexpensive fish roes on many supermarket shelves in the gourmet or canned fish aisle.

When to Call THE DOCTOR

It's a good idea to make a doctor's appointment when you first experience three or more consecutive days of wrist pain. Seeking help early can prevent permanent damage to the median nerve. You'll also want to rule out other painful conditions, such as arthritis, whose symptoms mimic carpal tunnel. If it is CTS, your doctor may suggest you wear a special splint and rest your wrist for a week or so. In advanced cases, you may require surgery.

Could it be an infection?

Recently, Australian hand surgeons wrote up a case report titled "An uncommon cause for a common complaint." Turns out that in rare cases, carpal tunnel syndrome can be caused by an infection. Known as infectious tenosynovitis, it comes in two forms. The gonococcal type is a sexually transmitted disease that commonly affects teenagers and young adults. The nongonococcal variety can occur following a puncture wound, cut, bite, or even a bout of dry, cracked skin. Sometimes, the wound can't even be found. So if your symptoms persist even after treatment and your doctor still can't pinpoint a cause, ask her to test you for this infection.

carpal tunnel syndrome

Add flaxseed to your cereal. Freshly ground flaxseed is extremely rich in plant-based omega-3 fatty acids, which reduce inflammation. Enjoy a couple of tablespoons every day in your yogurt, oatmeal, salad, or cereal—they add a nice nuttiness. Give it a couple of weeks to have an effect.

Use a spicy rub. The same kinds of remedies that ease arthritis pain may also ease CTS pain. One good choice is red pepper, which has a reputation as an arthritis remedy. Also known as cayenne, this spice contains a substance called capsaicin, which reduces the levels of the chemical compound substance P, which transmits pain signals to the brain. Mix a few dashes of ground cayenne pepper with 2 to 3 teaspoons olive oil. Apply with gauze to your wrist several times a day. Allow a week or more of continued use for the desensitization to take place. The first few doses will cause a mild, but usually tolerable burning sensation. Don't apply this remedy to inflamed or broken skin.

Find relief in the bathroom pantry. That pain-relieving capsaicin cream you bought the last time someone suffered a muscle ache or arthritis pain makes a great carpal tunnel treatment. Be sure to give it a few days to work.

Use bromelain. This protein-digesting enzyme derived from pineapple combats inflammation in the carpal tunnel from inside your body. Take 500 milligrams in supplement form when your stomach is empty (otherwise, it'll consume itself dissolving the food you've just eaten). It's easy to find in the vitamin aisle at the drugstore or in health food stores.

chapped lips

On anyone's list of health woes, chapped lips ranks way down at the bottom. But that doesn't mean they aren't annoying, irritating, and uncomfortable. Happily, many things can cure the problem, including some you can make at home from stuff that's right inside your pantry.

first things first

Prevention is easy when it comes to chapped lips: Just keep lip moisturizer in your purse or pocket. As soon as the weather gets cold and dry, treat your lips several times a day with a store-bought lip moisturizer or one of our recommended balms.

kitchen cabinet cures

Smooth on some honey. Plain honey is a great moisturizer. Apply some morning and night and just try not to lick it all off. Don't use honey on children under the age of one, because it may contain dangerous spores that infants' immune systems can't handle.

Squeeze out some vitamin E. Puncture a vitamin E capsule and apply the oil to your lips for some very healthy and effective relief.

Use shortening. When nothing better is at hand, olive oil or vegetable shortening, such as Crisco, will help to soften and moisturize chapped lips quite nicely. Just smooth directly on your lips.

Pantry HEALERS

Beeswax

Honey

Lavender
  essential oil

Olive oil

Tea tree essential oil

Vegetable
  shortening

Vitamin E capsules

Wintergreen
  essential oil

recipes for healing

Cocoa Lip Balm

Although this concoction smells tasty, it's not meant to be eaten. If you plan to give it to a child, label it accordingly and explain how to use it.

> ½ cup extra-virgin olive oil
> 1 tablespoon grated beeswax
> ½ teaspoon unsweetened cocoa powder
> 1 capsule vitamin E

1. In a microwave or the top of a double boiler, melt the oil and beeswax together. Do not boil. If the mixture starts to boil, remove from the heat and allow it to cool. Once the beeswax and oil are blended, stir in the cocoa powder. Pierce the vitamin E capsule with a needle, squeeze out half the contents, and stir it in. Pour the resulting mixture into clean containers with tops.

2. Let the lip balm sit for 48 hours at room temperature, or until it arrives at the proper consistency for spreading. You can carry a small container of lip balm around with you during the day, but you may find it keeps better in the refrigerator overnight.

Healing Lip Balm

If your lips are cracked and painful, this extra-soothing balm will help heal them before you know it.

> 4 tablespoons olive oil
> 1 tablespoon grated beeswax
> 1 teaspoon honey
> 1 capsule vitamin E
> 10 drops lavender essential oil
> 10 drops tea tree essential oil
> 10 drops wintergreen essential oil

1. In the top of a double boiler, warm the oil, beeswax, and honey over low heat until the wax melts. Remove from heat. Pierce the vitamin E capsule with a needle and squeeze its contents into the mixture.

2. Stir in the essential oils. Store in a cool, dark place and use by dipping a finger into the balm and smoothing it on your lips.

When to Call **THE DOCTOR**

Chapped lips usually clear up as soon as you moisturize them diligently. However, if you have chronically chapped lips, or if your lips regularly crack or bleed, see your doctor to rule out any medical conditions.

chicken pox

Chicken pox lasts only a week or two, but it can be a miserable time for little kids, especially when they're covered head to toe (and everyplace in between) with the spotty, itchy pox. And it can be an exhausting couple of weeks for moms and dads, too—this is one of those childhood illnesses that call for round-the-clock loving care. Even though the preventive vaccine may result in fewer children coming down with chicken pox, there will always be kids (and even some adults) who'll benefit from using these gentle kitchen pantry remedies in addition to the standard cures.

first things first

In addition to your arsenal of cures, take these actions the minute you know your child has chicken pox:

• If it's winter, turn down the heat to the lowest comfortable temperature. In summer, use air conditioning. Not available? Then put fans in your child's room. Heat brings more blood to the skin, which exacerbates the itch.

• Trim his or her fingernails as far back as you can, and keep them short. The goal is to make it as hard as possible to scratch open blisters. This helps prevent infection—and scarring.

• Offer your child a cool, wet washcloth to press against her skin when she feels like scratching. She'll be able to satisfy her urge to scratch but won't do any damage.

Pantry HEALERS

Bran flakes

Calamine lotion

Milk of magnesia

Oatmeal

Orange pekoe tea

Petroleum jelly

Salt

Tea tree essential oil

Shun the blistering sun

If your child has recently been exposed to someone with chicken pox, keep her out of the sun. A dose of sunshine may make the blisters worse when they finally erupt. After the chicken pox is over, your child's skin will remain sensitive to the sun for as long as a year. You don't have to barricade her in the house, but do apply sunscreen every day.

• For extra insurance against scratching, have your child wear cotton gloves to bed and clean, extra-soft, long-sleeve cotton pj's with long pants. Cotton is gentler to the skin than synthetic fabrics.

• Let your child get plenty of rest, and serve plenty of clear liquids and soft, bland foods, especially if there are sores in the mouth.

• Never give your child aspirin when she has chicken pox—or any other viral illness, for that matter. Doing so could cause Reye's syndrome, a complication that is potentially fatal.

kitchen cabinet cures

Go for an oatmeal swim. A nice cool (not cold) bath laced with a cup or so of baking soda or oatmeal will make your child feel much more comfortable. You can buzz a couple of handfuls of plain oatmeal in a food processor or blender and toss right in the tub. Or you can stuff finely ground oatmeal into a clean piece of panty hose and put that in the bathwater. Your child can use the oatmeal sock to rub gently on the pox.

Offer sips of orange pekoe tea. Home remedy advocates swear that drinking warm orange pekoe tea can speed the eruption of chicken pox sores—and the faster they emerge, the faster they'll dry up and heal. Sweeten with honey to make the tea more palatable. Don't use this for children under the age of one.

Dab on some milk of magnesia. Its soothing, drying action can work some magic on itchy pox.

Find the calamine lotion. Then swab onto the blisters. This pink lotion is made in large part of zinc oxide, which helps soothe and dry up the blisters.

Tap the tea tree. Blend a few drops of tea tree essential oil with 1 tablespoon of olive oil, and use a cotton swab to apply the oil to sores two or three times a day. Tea tree oil is a powerful natural antiseptic.

Prevent the crack-up. After sores have crusted over, coat them with some petroleum jelly to prevent them from cracking and bleeding. When you do this, however, make sure you don't transmit the virus to the stuff in the jar.

Instead of using your finger, apply the petroleum jelly with a cotton swab. Use a fresh swab every time.

Mind the mouth. If your child has chicken pox in his mouth (yes, it can happen), have him gargle with salt water. Serve soothing, bland foods like soups, gelatin, and bananas—items that won't hurt the blisters. Ice pops can also be soothing.

When to Call THE DOCTOR

Chicken pox is usually more of an annoyance than a danger; most cases clear up in 10 to 14 days without problems. Only in rare cases do serious complications emerge. Still, call your pediatrician once you suspect your child has chicken pox. The doctor can prescribe medications, if necessary, to lessen the severity of the disease. Seek immediate attention if your child has a high fever accompanied by severe headache, has a fever that lasts more than a few days, feels severe pain in his limbs, repeatedly vomits, develops a cough, or has a large area of warmth or redness surrounding one or more blisters—this is a sign of infection.

recipe for healing

Anti-itch Poultice

This poultice provides soothing relief for an itchy child. What's more, it contains that invisible ingredient—a mom or dad's loving touch—that makes it more powerful than any over-the-counter treatment you could ever buy.

> Water to cover
> 1 cup bran (pulverize plain bran flakes in the blender or food processor)

1. Boil the water and remove from heat.
2. Steep the bran in the water until it is room temperature. Strain, reserving the liquid.
3. Place the bran in a piece of cheesecloth and tie it securely so it's completely contained in the cloth.
4. Apply the bran bundle on the sores and let sit for 10 seconds, moving it from place to place until all the pox have been treated. Then rewet the bundle with the reserved bran water and repeat the application. Use the bran treatment every couple of hours for maximum relief.

cold sores

Canker sores might have many causes, but cold sores have just one: a particular type of herpes virus. And that's not the only difference between these mouth maladies. Canker sores mostly occur inside the mouth; cold sores usually appear on or around the lips. But in both cases, healing comes naturally and relatively quickly. And kitchen cabinet cures can help speed up and improve the process.

Pantry HEALERS

Aloe

Aspirin

B_{12} supplements

Black tea

Cornstarch

Lavender
  essential oil

Lemon balm
  essential oil

Lysine supplements

Olive oil

Red wine

Tea tree essential oil

first things first

Sometimes, you can prevent a cold sore from emerging—or reduce its severity—if you react quickly to the first sensations of one forming. Here's what to do:

• Apply a drop or two of lemon balm essential oil to the area as soon as you feel the tingle of a cold sore forming. Recent studies have proven that lemon balm essential oil effectively kills the herpes virus.

• Then hold an ice cube on top of the area for 10 minutes. Repeat the whole procedure several times a day.

kitchen cabinet cures

Dry up a little red wine. If you have an opened bottle of red wine handy, put a little bit in a saucer and let it sit until the liquid evaporates. Slather the sore with the solidified dregs and it will ease the pain on contact. Theory is that resveratrol, red wine's potent antioxidant, can relieve the inflammation. Despite the fact that experts say there's probably not enough resveratrol in wine dregs to make much of a difference, some folk healers swear by this trick.

Make a cornstarch paste. An old home remedy calls for making a cornmeal poultice for a cold sore. Here's an easier adaptation: Make a paste of a little cornstarch and water and dab it on the sore a few times a day. It will soothe and cool the inflammation.

Take lysine supplements. Along with lemon balm essential oil, this amino acid emerges as a hands-down best healer for cold sores. Take 3,000 milligrams daily until the sore goes away. Research shows it thwarts the replication of the virus.

Try a tea bag poultice. At the first twinge of a cold sore, apply a damp, cooled black tea bag to the area where you expect the outbreak to occur. Keep it on for 10 minutes. Repeat three or four times a day to reduce the duration and severity of an outbreak. It's been said that Earl Grey tea bags seem to be the most effective.

Beef up your B$_{12}$. Studies have shown that people who tend to get cold sores also tend to have low levels of vitamin B$_{12}$. Taking a daily B$_{12}$ supplement might lessen your chances for developing the sores.

Dab on some aloe. Cut off a little piece of your aloe plant, scrape off a bit of the gel, and swab the cold sore three or four times a day until the sore goes away.

Apply some tea tree oil. Apply tea tree essential oil directly on the cold sore three or four times a day.

Have an aspirin. It will offer you some pain relief. Research also shows that 125 milligrams of aspirin a day can cut the time a herpes infection remains active by 50 percent.

When to Call THE DOCTOR

If you have frequent bouts of cold sores, it could indicate a weakened immune system or that you're under undue stress that could be affecting your health in other ways. Check with your doctor to rule out medical causes, and ask her advice about ways to reduce your stress.

Weird & wacky

We found this one in a book about old home remedies: "To heal a cold sore quickly, put earwax on it." Naturally, we don't recommend the earwax treatment, though we do wonder what prompted its inventor to try it.

recipe for healing

Lemon Balm Cold Sore Treatment Oil
This recipe combines ingredients known to help heal cold sores. It also feels good on the sore.

> 5 drops lemon balm essential oil
> 2 drops lavender essential oil
> 10 drops olive oil

Blend the essential oils with the olive oil and dab on the sore three or four times a day.

colds & flu

Scientists studying the 99 known strains of rhinoviruses made a headline-worthy breakthrough in 2009. By decoding the viruses' genome, they discovered weaknesses they believe can finally lead to a cure for the common cold. The bad news is that cure is still a long way off. In the meantime, you can rely on trusted home remedies as your first line of defense against sniffling, sneezing, sore throat, coughing, and aches. These cures come right from your kitchen cabinet and help get you back on your feet fast.

first things first

There are certain hard-and-fast rules we should all follow when a cold or flu comes along. Among them:

- Stay home in a warm (but not overheated) room.
- Increase the moisture in the air with a humidifier if it makes you feel better (it won't speed your healing, though).
- Drink plenty of fluids.
- Get lots of rest.
- To keep the virus from spreading, cover your mouth when you sneeze or cough, and wash your hands frequently with soap and water.
- Do your friends, coworkers, and the public at large a favor by staying home until the symptoms pass.

Pantry HEALERS

Cayenne pepper

Elderberry

Eucalyptus
  essential oil

Flaxseeds

Garlic

Gingerroot

Honey

Lavender essential oil

Lemon

Mustard powder

Peppermint
  essential oil

Rubbing alcohol

Sage

Salt

Tea

Thyme

Witch hazel

Wintergreen
  essential oil

Zinc lozenges

kitchen cabinet cures

Eat garlic. There's no question that garlic boosts your immunity and fights viruses; researchers keep working to find just how effective it is. Though its effectiveness at easing colds is a matter of debate, herbalists often advise eating raw cloves at the onset of cold or flu symptoms (if you cook or dry garlic, it loses its antibiotic properties). To make it more palatable, chop up a clove of garlic and mix with a spoonful of honey, yogurt, or applesauce before eating. Chopping or crushing raw garlic activates its medicinal compounds.

Swallow a mustard-honey remedy. Mix ¼ teaspoon mustard powder with 2 tablespoons honey and swallow. This sweet-savory blend will help loosen chest congestion. Never give honey to babies under one year of age.

Try this wonderful tea. Put 5 slices of fresh gingerroot in a small saucepan and add 2 cups of water. Bring to boil, then simmer for 20 minutes. Drink the tea warm. The ginger is loaded with anti-inflammatory, germ-killing compounds. Make it even more delicious by adding some honey and orange juice. You'll get a shot of vitamin C from the OJ and a burst of soothing antiseptic power from the honey.

Breathe in these spices. Aromatic, germ-killing herbs and humidity can do wonders for a stuffed-up head. This treatment takes only minutes to put together, and the

When to Call THE DOCTOR

If you're sidelined with a miserable cold, especially if it's accompanied by a fever and aching, call your doctor's office even if you think it's "just a cold." You'll learn about any flu hitting the community, and your doctor's office will suggest the best course of action. Generally, they'll want to see you in person if a fever lasts for more than three days or if your temperature is over 102°F. Never give aspirin to a child with a virus; this increases the risk of Reye's syndrome, a rare but life-threatening disease.

Is sweating healing?

You'd certainly think so, since so many home remedies, like mustard plasters and steaming cups of ginger tea, make you perspire. These remedies have their place: Mustard plasters can help break up chest congestion, and ginger tea lowers fevers and kills cold viruses.

But you can't get rid of a cold by simply sweating it out—unless you're working up that sweat by exercising. Turns out, hopping on a treadmill or getting some other form of aerobic exercise gives you a little relief. It opens up sinuses and allows them to drain. And according to doctors at the Mayo Clinic, exercising gives you a shot of a natural cold-fighting drug, adrenalin. Chemically related to all the drugs used to treat cold symptoms, adrenalin levels go up when you exercise. What's more, when researchers asked people with colds to work out on treadmills, they learned that their colds didn't limit their ability to exercise.

results are priceless. Put 1 tablespoon each of dried thyme, sage, and peppermint into a medium bowl and add boiling water. Lean over the bowl with a towel draped over your head, close your eyes, and inhale for 10 minutes. For safety, keep your face at least 10 inches above the water. Repeat two or three times a day as needed.

Use saline spray for clogged sinuses. Breathe easier quickly by thoroughly mixing ¼ teaspoon table salt into 1 cup of boiled water. Let cool until it's a comfortably warm temperature. To get the solution into your nose, use an ear bulb syringe (like the kind used to clean out a baby's nose), a neti pot (an Indian sinus-cleaning tool available in health food stores), or a water pick(also know as an oral irrigator) on the lowest setting (you'll need a special adapter for this). Flush your nasal passages two or three times a day.

Find some zinc lozenges. Zinc gluconate lozenges are among the top remedies for colds and flu. In one study, people who sucked on a lozenge containing about

|||||||||||||||||||||||||||||||||||||||||||||||||||||||||||||||||||||||||||||||||||||||||||||||||||||||||||||||||||||||||||||||||||||||||||||||||||||||||

Soup's on!

We're hard-pressed to think of a country that doesn't have its own version of Mom's chicken soup. From Mexico to China and ports of call in between, mothers serve up bowls of the fragrant liquid whenever their loved ones come down with cold and flu miseries. In some circles, it's known as "Jewish penicillin," and in fact, studies show that hot chicken soup seems to be more effective at clearing nasal passages than other hot liquids are. Somehow, chicken soup inhibits the movement of white blood cells, which contributes to inflammation of the lining of the respiratory tract. And, of course, it offers plenty of nutrition and fluids—and if you're lucky, a dumpling or noodles and some soft vegetables.

For greater healing power, add chopped garlic to your chicken soup. But be sure to toss it in just before you serve it, because heat destroys garlic's medicinal compounds. Also consider spiking your chicken soup with a dash of red pepper sauce, red pepper flakes, or wasabi, the condiment (usually made from horseradish) that's eaten with sushi. All of these red-hot add-ins can increase the broth's decongestant power. In fact, adding any of them to any food can help you breathe more freely.

Other hot beverages also have a place in your cold-healing arsenal. Hot lemonade, like any hot drink, decreases congestion (although the effect is short-lived), and it also provides a healthy dose of vitamin C, which may help fight off colds and lessen their severity. Tea with honey also helps break up congestion and soothes a sore throat. Herb teas made with sage and thyme have germ-killing properties and can decrease inflammation.

13 milligrams of zinc every two hours while awake, shook off their symptoms three to four days sooner than people who didn't. Just don't take them continuously for more than a week.

While you're at it, grab some elderberry. At the first sign of the flu, take an elderberry syrup called Sambucol. Elderberry has been used in Europe for centuries to fight viruses. One lab study showed that Sambucol killed 10 flu strains, and in a human study, it reduced flu recovery time to three or four days. More recently, in a test tube study conducted at a Florida research lab, elderberry extract killed the H1N1 virus. Another option: elderberry flower tea. Make it by putting 10 elderberry tea bags in a quart canning jar filled with just-boiled water. Cover and steep for 20 minutes. Sweeten with honey to taste. Drink one cup every four hours, reheating the tea when necessary. Elderberry flower products are sold in health food stores.

Attack with pepper spray. This is a classic case of fighting fire with fire—and it works like a charm to ease sore throat pain. In a clean 8-ounce spray bottle, combine

Elderberry is emerging as one of the world's top flu remedies.

||||||||||||||||||||||||||||||||||||||||||||||||||||||||||||||||||||||||||||||||||||||||||||||||||||||||||||||||||||||||||||||||||||

Cold or flu: an update

Both colds and flu are caused by viruses. There are many more cold viruses than strains of the flu, but they are relatively minor infections. Cold viruses primarily inflame the mucous membranes that line your nose and throat. The all-too-familiar symptoms include a runny nose, sneezing, watery eyes, and sometimes a sore throat, aches, and coughing. Most colds clear up within a week or so.

Influenza is a more serious illness. It usually brings with it fever, chills, muscle aches, and sometimes back pain, in addition to cold symptoms. The flu typically comes on suddenly and can lead to secondary infections, such as bronchitis and pneumonia, which require much more serious medical treatment. For that reason, the flu can pose a serious health threat, especially to the elderly.

Flu viruses are notorious shape shifters. The most recent flu incarnation, the H1N1, is sweeping its way around the world. This strain has proven to be dangerous to otherwise healthy young people, as well as to pregnant women and people with chronic conditions like asthma and diabetes. If you've been exposed to the flu or suspect you may be coming down with it, see your doctor right away. He or she can prescribe drugs called Tamiflu or Relenza, which can stop the flu virus from spreading through your body. Taking one of these drugs can lessen flu symptoms and shorten their duration. They may also be able to prevent the flu once you've been exposed.

1 tablespoon of cayenne pepper with just enough water to almost fill the bottle. Shake well and use as a spray to numb the back of your throat. You can also use the mix as a gargle. Just don't get it near your eyes.

Lap up some lemon. The traditional sore-throat gargle—a squeeze of lemon juice in a glass of hot water—works because it creates an acidic environment that's hostile to bacteria and viruses.

Stir up some honey and lemon tea. There's something about this simple throat-soothing tea that makes you feel nurtured when you're fighting a cold. And it's remarkably effective. The honey soothes and coats your throat and is a natural antiseptic. The lemon acts as an astringent, shrinking swollen throat tissue.

Bare-cupboard throat fix. Even if your pantry is empty, you've got these two ingredients on hand—and they work remarkably well. Just fill an 8-ounce glass with warm water, mix in 1 teaspoon salt, and gargle away. The salt really does soothe the pain.

Cut short a cold with your...blow-dryer. As crazy as it sounds, inhaling heated air may help kill a virus working its way up your nose. In one study conducted at Harvard Hospital in England, people who breathed heated air had half the cold symptoms of people who inhaled air at room temperature. Set your hair dryer on warm (not hot), hold it at least 18 inches from your face, and breathe in the air through your nose for as long as you can—at least 2 or 3 minutes, and preferably 20 minutes.

recipes for healing

Minty Chest Rub
This homemade chest rub can relax you and calm your cough.

> 12 drops eucalyptus essential oil
> 4 drops peppermint essential oil
> 2 tablespoons olive oil or vegetable oil

1. In a small dish, mix the eucalyptus and peppermint essential oils with the olive oil.
2. Rub the mixture onto your chest and cover with a damp, warm towel (try warming the damp towel in the microwave). Leave on until the warmth fades.

Simple Mustard Powder Plaster
This mustard plaster produces heat without being hot to the touch. Mixing water with the powdered seed forms a volatile oil which irritates (and can burn) the skin, increasing blood flow. When using a mustard plaster, do not let the skin become too red. To soothe any burning, wash the area with cold water. Protect the skin beforehand by applying petroleum jelly to the area. To make a milder plaster, use less mustard powder or replace the water with milk or an egg. Do not leave on longer than 10 to 15 minutes.

> 1 tablespoon mustard powder
> 2 tablespoons all-purpose flour

1. In a bowl, mix the mustard powder with the flour. Add enough water to make a paste.
2. Spread the paste over half of a dish towel. Fold the towel in half, covering the paste, and apply to the chest. Don't apply the mustard paste directly onto the skin. Check the chest skin often and remove the mustard plaster if there are signs of irritation.

Nighttime Breathing Relief
Getting a good night's sleep is probably the best thing you can do for a cold. This recipe allows you to breathe so you can sleep through the night. The key oil in this formula is eucalyptus; you can triple the amount you use if you omit the other two oils.

> 2–4 drops peppermint essential oil
> 2–4 drops eucalyptus essential oil
> 2–4 drops wintergreen essential oil

1. In a small bowl, mix the oils together. Dip a cotton ball into the mixture and put it near the vent of a steam humidifier.
2. Place the humidifier and the cotton ball near your bed when you have a cold.

Extra-Strength Mustard Plaster

This recipe makes a slightly thicker, stronger mustard plaster. Do not leave on longer than 30 minutes.

> 2 tablespoons or more olive oil
> ¹/₃ cup yellow mustard seeds
> 2 tablespoons grated beeswax

1. Put 2 tablespoons olive oil and the mustard seeds into a blender and blend. Continue adding olive oil until you have a thick liquid.

2. Pour the mixture into the top of a double boiler over low heat; add the beeswax and heat, stirring, until the wax melts. Spread a dish towel on a flat surface. Once the mustard-wax mixture is warm and can be spread, apply it to the towel and let it cool to room temperature.

3. Place the towel salve-side-down on the chest and cover with a T-shirt or old flannel, then apply external heat on top with a heating pad or hot-water bottle. You should start to feel warmth seeping into your chest in about 10 to 15 minutes. Leave it on another 15 minutes. You can store the plaster in the fridge for several days; when needed, remove and let it warm to room temperature before using.

Flaxseed Toddy

This old farmers' remedy is said to be a good cold cure. At the very least, it's hot, tasty, and soothing.

> 2 ounces flaxseeds
> 2 ounces sugar
> 1 cup honey
> Juice of 3 lemons

1. Boil the flaxseeds in 1 quart of water for 5 to 10 minutes. Strain out the flaxseeds.

2. Add the sugar, honey, and lemon to the hot water and blend.

3. Drink ½ cup before meals and a cup at bedtime. Refrigerate the remaining toddy, but heat before using.

Herbal Inhalant

Make this soothing breathing reliever and tote it along to help ease congestion.

> ¼ to ½ teaspoon rock salt
> 2–4 drops peppermint essential oil
> 2–4 drops eucalyptus essential oil
> 2–4 drops wintergreen essential oil

1. Put the rock salt in the bottom of a small glass bottle or jar with a tight-fitting lid. Add the oils.

2. Carry with you and sniff as needed to open clogged nasal passages.

Decongestant Salve

This rub can give that expensive stuff from the pharmacy a run for its money.

> ½ cup olive oil
>
> 1 tablespoon peppermint essential oil
>
> 1 tablespoon eucalyptus essential oil
>
> 1 tablespoon wintergreen essential oil
>
> ½ ounce grated beeswax
>
> 4 drops tincture of benzoin (available at drugstores)

1. In the top of a double boiler over low heat, heat the olive oil and the essential oils. Add the beeswax and tincture of benzoin and stir until the beeswax is melted and the oils are well mixed.

2. Pour the mixture into a clean, wide-mouthed jar with a tight-fitting lid and allow to cool. Put under your nose or rub on your chest as a decongestant. You can keep this mixture, covered, in a cool, dark place for up to two weeks. Wash your hands after applying so you don't accidentally get any salve in your eyes.

Sore Throat Gargle

This old-fashioned gargle will soothe a sore throat, and the sweetness may tempt kids to gargle a little longer.

> 2 heaping tablespoons brown sugar
>
> ½ teaspoon salt
>
> ¼ teaspoon baking soda
>
> 2 cups warm water

1. In a jar with a tight-fitting lid, combine the brown sugar, salt, baking soda, and warm water. Shake well before each use.

2. Gargle with up to ½ cup four times a day as needed. Make a fresh batch each day.

Fever-Relief Spray

Spraying pulse points with a cool, soothing solution might help lower a fever. At the very least, spritzing on this refreshing blend will soothe you and make you feel more comfortable. The pulse points are the places on the body where you can easily feel your heart rate when you touch them with your fingers—typically inside your wrists, just under each side of the jaw, and the back of the knees.

> ¼ cup rubbing alcohol or vodka
>
> ¼ cup witch hazel
>
> 3 drops peppermint essential oil
>
> 2 drops lavender essential oil

1. In a clean spray bottle, combine the rubbing alcohol, witch hazel, and peppermint and lavender oils. Shake to mix and then chill in the refrigerator.

2. Spray onto pulse points to reduce fever, avoiding your eyes and mouth.

constipation

Feeling "all backed up" is uncomfortable in so many ways. There's the bloated feeling, the unproductive straining, and the insecurity of knowing that you might suddenly need to let go at a most inopportune time. Constipation can have a slew of causes, including a fiber-poor diet, not drinking enough fluids, stress, laxative dependence, lack of exercise, and certain prescription drugs or health conditions. As luck would have it, constipation also has a slew of solutions, many of which can be found right in your kitchen pantry.

first things first

Here are the basic approaches to start with when things just don't seem to be moving the right way:

• The best way to become "regular" again is simply to eat more fiber—20 to 35 grams a day. Fiber absorbs water and makes your stool softer and larger, which speeds it through your system.

• To cope with all that fiber, you'll need more fluids too. Drink more water than usual.

• And don't forget about exercise, which can also help keep things moving.

• When you feel the urge, head to the bathroom. If you "put it off till later," you're asking for a case of constipation.

• On the other hand, don't try to force a bowel movement. You may give yourself hemorrhoids or anal fissures. These not only hurt, they aggravate constipation.

Pantry HEALERS

Coffee

Corn syrup

Epsom salts

Figs

Flaxseeds

Honey

Lemon

Prunes

Psyllium seeds

Raisins

Sesame seeds

Tea

kitchen cabinet cures

Fix up a flax drink. Boil a couple of cups of water with 2 tablespoons flaxseeds. Strain and cool, then add a teaspoon of apple cider vinegar and drink. The fiber and liquid combo can help move things along.

Open some sesames. An Amish remedy for constipation—and one espoused by Chinese folk healers—is sesame seeds. Their oily composition helps moisturize the intestines, which can help if dry stools are a problem. Spin ½ ounce of the tasty seeds in a clean coffee grinder and sprinkle on food like a seasoning.

Syrup trick for infants. If your baby is constipated, add 1 teaspoon of corn syrup to 4 ounces of water or formula. It can work as a stool softener and make stools easier to pass.

Pop some psyllium. The seeds of a plantain relative, psyllium, is the laxative most recommended by modern herbalists and doctors. It can also be an effective treatment for irritable bowel syndrome and hemorrhoids. Though it's probably not something you'll find in your kitchen cabinet, you may want to run out to the health food store to pick some up. Relief is very likely to follow. Add 2 teaspoons of the seeds to a little water and let them swell slightly. Take in the morning and at night with 1 or 2 glasses of fluid. Although rare, allergic reactions or intestinal obstruction may occur.

When to Call THE DOCTOR

Chronic constipation can signal serious conditions, colorectal cancer and bowel obstruction among them. Tell your doctor if the problem lasts two weeks or more despite using the remedies in this chapter. Call your doctor immediately if you see blood in your stool or if constipation is accompanied by fever, severe abdominal pain, cramps, or unexplained weight loss. Also, if you've recently started a new medication that seems to cause constipation, advise your doctor. Possible drug culprits include antihistamines, diuretics, blood-pressure drugs, sedatives, calcium supplements, certain antidepressants, and antacids that contain calcium or aluminum.

Lay off the laxatives

Stimulant laxatives can be addictive, and using them regularly can lead to loss of important nutrients and permanent loss of bowel control. Even worse, their abuse has been linked to colon cancer. If you're dieting, you might be taking these unwittingly, because stimulant laxatives can be hidden in over-the-counter weight loss teas and supplements. Avoid diet aids that contain senna leaf (*Cassia senna*), cascara sagrada bark (*Rhamnus purshiana*), or castor oil.

Not all laxatives are dangerous, however. The bulk-producing laxatives, such as Metamucil, contain psyllium seed husks. This natural substance absorbs liquid in the intestines, swells up, and naturally triggers the urge to move the bowels. Other safe choices are the emollient laxatives, or stool softeners. They allow water or fat to penetrate the stool, or they help lay down a smooth coating that lets stools pass easier. Examples include Colace, mineral oil, and glycerin suppositories.

Get-up-and-go

There's a reason a daily walk is called a constitutional. When you move your body, you also help move food through your bowel more quickly. Aim for a 15-minute daily walk at the very least. The more you move, the more you "move."

Drink coffee to loosen up. If you're a java drinker, you may have already discovered that the caffeine in coffee has a bowel-loosening effect. It induces a bowel movement by stimulating the colon. Just don't drink too much of it—caffeine is a diuretic and will eliminate fluid from your body.

Or try other hot drinks. If you don't like coffee, try any other hot beverage first thing in the morning. Herbal or decaffeinated tea or a cup of hot water with a little lemon juice or honey may stimulate the colon as well. (Lemon juice is a natural laxative.)

Grab some prunes. The number one classic kitchen remedy for getting bowels back on track is fiber-rich prunes. (Three prunes contain 3 grams of fiber.) What's more, a prune compound called dihydroxyphenyl isatin helps trigger the intestinal contractions that make you want to go. An old grandmother's remedy for

IIIIIIIIIIIIIIIIIIIIIIIIIIIIIIIIIIIIIIIIIIIIIIIIIIIIIIIIIIIIIIIIIIIIIIIIIIIIIIIIIII

Kitchen cabinet fiber foods

If you're wondering how to get more fiber in your diet for better regularity, look to these kitchen pantry staples, all excellent sources of fiber.

Food	Portion size	Fiber Grams
Bran cereal	½ cup	10–14
Red kidney beans	½ cup	8.2
Shredded Wheat'n Bran cereal	1¼ cups	7.9
Lentils, boiled	1½ cups	7.8
Black beans	½ cup	7.5
Figs, dried	3	6.9
Navy beans	½ cup	6.7
Whole-wheat spaghetti, cooked	1 cup	6.3
Pinto beans	½ cup	5.5
Oatmeal, cooked	1 cup	5.0
Green split-pea soup	1 cup	5.0
Almonds	1 ounce	3.3
Prunes, canned	5	3.3
Pearl barley	½ cup	3.0
Dates	5	3.0
Prunes, dried	5	3.0

constipation: Soak a handful of prunes in boiled water overnight. First thing in the morning, drink the water, then eat the soaked prunes. Another great dried fruit choice is figs, which will get your move on and may not cause as much bloating as prunes can.

Reach for raisins. Raisins are also high in fiber and contain tartaric acid, which has a laxative effect. In one study in which people ate 4½ ounces (one small box) of raisins a day, doctors determined that it took half the time for digested food to make it through the digestive tract.

Stir up some honey and lemon. Try having a cup of hot water mixed with a tablespoon of lemon or lime juice and a tablespoon of honey. The juice stimulates the release of bile, and that can kick-start intestinal contractions.

Get out the salts. Since its discovery in a mineral spring in the village of Epsom, England, in 1695, Epsom salts have been a popular constipation remedy. They work because they draw water into the intestines, and that's what enables bowel flow. To use, stir 2 or 3 teaspoons into a glass of warm water and drink in the morning. Don't use this remedy for more than seven days—it can cause dehydration and laxative dependence.

coughs

You're coughing so hard that the floor is shaking. Your chest hurts, you're keeping yourself and your family awake at night, and you're utterly miserable. Though it feels absolutely awful, a bad cough is actually a good thing. It's part of your body's sophisticated defense system and helps rid the respiratory tract of phlegm. Coughs can be caused by a cold, influenza, bronchitis, or pneumonia. Dust or smoke can trigger a dry cough—as can a case of nerves. In all cases, there are plenty of options for quick, soothing relief.

first things first

When you have a cough, there are basic steps to follow, in addition to trying the following remedies:

• Of course, cover your mouth when you cough. And then wash your hands frequently (consider keeping a bottle of hand sanitizer next to you until you get better).

• Drink plenty of liquids, especially hot tea. Coughing can be dehydrating; hot tea not only replenishes your fluid levels, but relieves your throat.

• Let yourself cough, particularly if it's productive (meaning it is bringing up phlegm). That means not taking cough suppressants.

• If your cough is productive, speed up the healing process by inhaling lots of steam, either from a vaporizer, shower, or steam treatment. It'll help break up and expel the congestion.

kitchen cabinet cures

Pick some thyme. Thyme is an officially approved German treatment for coughs, upper respiratory infections, bronchitis, and whooping cough, with good reason. Those tiny leaves are packed with cough-relieving compounds. For starters, thyme flavonoids relax tracheal and ileal muscles, which are involved in coughing. The flavonoids also reduce inflammation. To make a tea, mix 2 teaspoons crushed leaves in 1 cup boiling water, cover, then steep for 10 minutes and strain.

Fight back with flax, honey, and lemon. Boiling flaxseeds in water gives you a thick, gooey gel that soothes the throat and the bronchial tract. Honey and lemon act as mild antibiotics and make this syrup super-soothing. To make it, boil 2 to 3 tablespoons of flaxseeds in 1 cup of water until the water becomes thick. Strain, then add 3 tablespoons each of honey and lemon juice. Take 1 tablespoon as needed.

Brew black pepper tea. This remedy is rooted in two very different traditions: New England folk medicine and traditional Chinese medicine. The rationale behind it is that black pepper stimulates circulation and mucus flow; honey is a natural cough reliever and mild antibiotic. To make the tea, place 1 teaspoon of freshly ground black pepper and 2 tablespoons of honey in a cup. Fill with boiling water and let steep, covered, for 15 minutes. Strain and sip as needed. This remedy works best on coughs that produce mucus and isn't suitable for dry coughs.

Another sour approach. This isn't for the feint of heart, but it is a commonly used folk cure: Quarter a fresh lemon, sprinkle it with lots of black pepper and salt, and suck on it for quick relief.

Try some warm milk. Another popular folk cure for a cough is to drink a cup of hot milk sweetened with honey.

Consider almonds. Some ancient traditions believe almonds help relieve bronchial problems, including coughs. They recommend blending a few teaspoons of finely ground almonds with a cup of orange juice and sipping it for relief.

When to Call THE DOCTOR

If you have difficulty breathing or swallowing, have thick greenish-yellow or bloody phlegm, a fever, stiff neck, or wheezing, see your doctor. Call 911 if you can't catch your breath or if your face swells and you have hives. Finally, check in with your doctor if an otherwise uncomplicated cough lasts longer than two weeks.

the natural DOCTOR'S Rx

Believe it or not, rinsing your nasal passages with a mild saline solution can ease your cough. That's because coughs are often caused or worsened by postnasal drip. Spritzing the inside of your nose helps wash out mucus that would otherwise drip, drip, drip down your throat. Here's how: Make a saline solution with ¼ teaspoon salt and ¼ teaspoon baking soda in 8 ounces of warm water. Place the saline solution in a neti pot (a little container made exactly for this purpose and found at health food stores). Or you can also use a small plastic bottle with a nasal tip, or even a water pick (also known as an oral irrigator) fitted with a special nasal tip.

recipes for healing

Lemony Cough Syrup

This tasty formula works brilliantly to ease coughs. Both honey and lemon are antibacterial, and the honey is soothing. What's more, it's scientifically proven to work. Researchers at Pennsylvania State University studied 105 coughing kids who received buckwheat honey, a honey-flavored preparation containing dextromethorphan (the ingredient in many cough syrups), or no treatment at all. Parents reported that kids who got honey saw the greatest reduction in coughing severity and frequency. Never give honey to children under the age of one. It's not safe for them.

> 1 lemon
> 1 pint raw honey

1. In a small saucepan, cover the whole lemon in water and simmer for 5 minutes.
2. In a separate saucepan, warm the honey, but don't let it boil. A slow cooker works perfectly.
3. Remove the lemon from the pan and wait until it's cool enough to handle, then slice it and add it to the honey. Let the honey and lemon cook on warm heat for an hour—do not allow to boil.
4. Cool, then strain into a sterilized jar and refrigerate. Have a teaspoon of the syrup whenever you need cough relief.

Super Onion Cough Syrup

After honey, lemon, and whiskey, onion is the ingredient most commonly included in cough remedies. Turns out, there are two good reasons why. First, onions relieve inflammation that can reduce irritation. And they contain a substance called protocatechuic acid that attacks viruses, like the one that may be causing your cough.

> 5 or 6 onions
> ½ cup honey
> Juice of 1 lemon

1. Chop the onions and place them in the top of a double boiler.
2. Add the honey and lemon and cook over very low heat for 3 or 4 hours.
3. Strain and take a tablespoon or two as needed.

Steam Cough Relief

This herbal steam treatment is a triple threat against coughs. First, the steam opens up breathing passages and thins mucus, making it easier to expel. Thyme reduces spasms in muscles that control coughing, and eucalyptus kills many of the bacteria that cause bacterial respiratory infections, plus it reduces bronchial inflammation.

4 cups water

3 tablespoons dried thyme

5 drops eucalyptus essential oil

1. In a saucepan over medium heat, heat the water until nearly boiling (but don't boil). Pour into a heat-safe bowl and add the thyme and eucalyptus oil.

2. Hold your head about 8 inches above the water, drape a towel over your head and the bowl to make a tent, and breathe in deeply until the water cools. Keep your eyes closed throughout.

Herbal Steam Treatment for Congestion

Aromatic herbs and humidity can do wonders easing coughs and chest congestion. This treatment takes only minutes to put together, and it's heavenly to use.

I tablespoon dried thyme, chopped

I tablespoon dried sage, chopped

I tablespoon dried peppermint, chopped

Boiling water

1. Put the thyme, sage, and peppermint in a medium bowl and add boiling water.

2. Let steep for a minute.

3. Lean over the bowl with a towel draped over your head and the bowl and inhale for 10 minutes. Keep your face 8 to 10 inches above the steaming water. Repeat two or three times a day as needed.

diarrhea

There's nothing subtle about diarrhea. A bout of loose bowels can overtake you suddenly, out of the blue. The siege can resolve quickly or linger for days and will certainly disrupt your life as long as it lasts—chances are, you'll be going nowhere until it abates. Common causes include food poisoning, a change in eating habits, or traveling to countries where foreign water and foods disagree with you. Viral, bacterial, or even parasitic infections could also be to blame, as can stress. Happily, most cases are minor and pass quickly, and several handy items from your kitchen cabinet can contribute to a speedier recovery.

first things first

Here's the immediate response you should have to the arrival of diarrhea:

• Resist that urge to run to the drugstore for an over-the-counter anti-diarrhea medicine. Diarrhea is your body's defense mechanism against noxious substances, so let yourself purge before you put a stop to the process.

• While you're under siege, keep eating to a minimum, and drink plenty of fluids. Best are electrolyte drinks like Gatorade, which can restore fluids and help prevent dehydration.

kitchen cabinet cures

Sip clear broth or juice. Apple juice and clear broth will help replace salts and minerals lost to diarrhea. But avoid citrus, pineapple, tomato, and other juices that you can't see through because the acid in them can irritate already inflamed intestines. Start with small sips and work your way up to drinking a cup every half hour.

Sip orange peel tea. A traditional diarrhea remedy and general digestive aid, orange peels stimulate digestion. You need organic oranges for this brew; nonorganic orange skins may contain dyes and pesticides. Peel an orange and chop the peel finely. Place in a pot and cover with a pint of boiling water. Cover the pot tightly and steep till cool. Strain, sweeten with honey, and drink.

Calm yourself with chamomile. This tea, known for its gentle relaxation powers, can also calm bouts of diarrhea. It attacks the problem on two fronts, via compounds that ease intestinal spasms and combat inflammation. To brew, use two chamomile tea bags per cup of boiled water. Let steep, covered, for 15 minutes. Drink a cup three times a day while you're under the weather.

Sip some vinegar water. If a bacterial infection is at the root of your diarrhea, apple cider vinegar could help contain the problem, thanks to its antibiotic properties. What's more, some folk remedy experts contend that apple cider vinegar contains pectin, which can help soothe intestinal spasms.

Offer caraway tea. To calm the intestinal spasms and discomfort that accompany diarrhea, try sipping caraway tea. Brew it by adding a teaspoon of caraway seeds to a cup of boiling water, cover, and let steep for 15 minutes. Strain through a fine sieve before serving.

Or try these other teas. Tannins in black tea have an astringent action on the mucous membranes in the intestines. This helps the body absorb fluids and calms intestinal inflammation. In particular, blackberry and raspberry leaf teas are praised by herbalists for their ability to ease diarrhea. Be sure to choose teas made from real leaves (some berry teas are mainly flavoring). Choose decaffeinated black teas; caffeine is dehydrating. (There is no caffeine in herbal teas.) Red teas, such as rooibos, can calm spasms in the colon.

Bind yourself up with rice. Plain white rice is known for its "binding effect" on bowels. Eat small portions of white rice, butter-free, until diarrhea is under control.

When to Call THE DOCTOR

Call your doctor if your diarrhea lasts more than 24 hours. And if you have any of these symptoms, call your doctor right away or seek emergency care:

• Pain, fever, or the presence of blood or mucous in the stool

• Persistent diarrhea or an inability to diagnose the diarrhea's cause

• A sense of becoming dehydrated (symptoms of this include constant thirst, dark-colored urine, dry mouth, fatigue, weakness, or chills)

the natural DOCTOR'S ℞

Friendly bacteria—often called probiotics and which include well-known types like acidophilus—are great for helping resolve diarrhea. You can find probiotics in yogurt that contains "live active cultures," or you can buy them in supplement form at drugstores and health food stores. Read yogurt labels to be sure the ones you choose contain high numbers of several strains of these good bugs, and stick with plain or vanilla nonfat yogurt while you're ill.

As to food, stick to the tried-and-true BRAT diet while your bowels are under siege: bananas, plain rice, applesauce, dry toast, and tea.

Honey to the rescue. Many cultures swear by honey as a cure for diarrhea. Mix 4 tablespoons of honey into a cup of hot water. Let cool and drink. It's very sweet, but effective.

Try some applesauce. Applesauce contains pectin, which helps to firm soft bowel movements. Consider applesauce spread on a slice of toast. But avoid apple juice—it contains little pectin and could make the situation worse.

Consider this ancient approach. Many cultures swear by buttermilk as a diarrhea remedy. An Ayurvedic healing approach is to mix ½ teaspoon of dry ginger into a cup of buttermilk and drink that three to four times a day.

 recipes for healing

DIY Electrolyte Drink

This simple formula helps maintain your body's equilibrium.

> 1 cup apple juice
> 2 cups water
> 1 teaspoon salt
> Juice from a lemon or a lime

1. In a pitcher, combine apple juice, water, salt, and the lemon or lime juice. Store in the refrigerator.
2. Drink throughout the day to maintain hydration and proper balance of electrolytes.

Pantry Rehydrator

Sip this solution all day long to make sure you're replenishing fluids flushed by diarrhea. Drink up to 3 quarts a day.

> ½ teaspoon salt
> ½ teaspoon baking soda
> 4 tablespoons sugar
> 1 liter of water

Mix all ingredients in a pitcher until dissolved and drink as needed.

earache

Ears are prone to problems that make them hurt. Blame it on their delicate architecture. Inside your ear, the moist, dark, narrow canals that loop-di-loop like a snail's shell are ideal harbors for bacteria. While young children are most prone to earaches, they're not the only ones who suffer from their pain; ear infections can strike at any age. Plus water enthusiasts of any age can contract swimmer's ear (otitis externa), the ear canal infection caused when bacteria invade the skin that lines the canal. Fortunately, there are easy ways to deal with most earaches, and they all start with ingredients found in your pantry.

first things first

• Don't race to the doctor the minute an earache strikes. These days, most docs recommend taking a 72-hour "wait-and-see" approach—both for grownups and kids (as long as your baby is otherwise healthy and her symptoms are mild). Since most cases of otitis media (the official name for inner ear infections) clear up on their own, waiting it out can prevent the overuse of antibiotics.

• Apply a warm, moist cloth over the ear to help relieve pain.

• Take a mild over-the-counter pain reliever to reduce the pain. If it's a child with the earache, ask his or her doctor first before giving pain medicine.

Pantry HEALERS

Apple cider vinegar

Garlic

Olive oil

Peppermint essential oil

Salt

Sesame oil

Vodka

Xylitol gum

Surprise! An ingredient in sugar-free gum helps prevent ear infections.

kitchen cabinet cures

Shake up the Italian salt trick. Heat a cup or so of coarse salt in a pan till hot. Put the heated salt in a thick cotton sock (using a funnel makes this easier) and tie the end. Test against your inner wrist to make sure it's not too hot, then hold the sock against your child's hurting ear. At the very least, the warmth will ease discomfort. And it's also possible that the salt will draw fluid from the infection, which theoretically could relieve middle ear pressure.

Put vinegar to work. Mix 2 tablespoons apple cider vinegar with 2 tablespoons warm water and put it in a dropper bottle. Instill four drops in the painful ear four times a day.

Harness the healing power of vodka. Try putting three drops of room-temperature vodka in a painful ear to relieve pain and help kill bacteria.

Make a salty gargle. Gargling with warm salt water when ear pain begins can help some children. The liquid's heat increases the flow of blood to the eustachian tubes, which link the ears and throat.

Xylitol gum to the rescue. The sweetener xylitol, which comes from birch trees and is also found in strawberries and plums, cuts down the growth of bacteria that cause middle-ear infections. In one study, children who chewed two pieces of the gum five times a day for two months had 40 percent fewer ear infections. Trident chewing gum is one of several brands that contain xylitol.

Open sesame (oil). If you cook Asian cuisine, you probably have a bottle of sesame oil in your pantry. Turns out it is a popular folk remedy for earaches. Add half a clove of

Remove wax safely

To remove earwax, put 10 drops of hydrogen peroxide in each ear and let it stay there for three minutes. Then tilt the head so the liquid runs out—and the wax with it. Never, ever try to excavate wax with cotton swabs, paper clips, hair pins, or similar tools. Granny's advice is still best: Never stick anything smaller than your elbow in your ear.

garlic to a teaspoon of sesame oil and heat until warm. Lie on your side and put four drops into the painful ear. Leave it in for 10 minutes, then drain.

Or try olive oil. Many folk healers say that olive oil is an effective earache remedy. As with sesame oil, heat until warm, then put about four drops into your ear. Let sit for 10 minutes, then drain.

Use peppermint. A similar remedy from days gone by is peppermint essential oil. Thoroughly blend one drop of peppermint oil with 20 drops of olive oil and put four drops of the mix in the infected ear. Drain after 10 minutes. Other old-timers say to apply the peppermint oil around the outside of your ear. Just make sure pure peppermint oil never enters your ear.

When to Call THE DOCTOR

Ear pain isn't usually an emergency. If it's a baby with the earache, see the doctor if the pain seems extreme or the child has a fever over 100°F. As for you, call the doctor if the pain doesn't go away after two days. Tell the doctor about any fluid discharge from the ear, dizziness, or painful sensations when you chew. Sudden, intense pain, followed by some relief, could indicate a ruptured eardrum. Other common signs of ruptured eardrum are discharge (sometimes with blood), muffled hearing, a ringing in the ears, and a feeling of dizziness or vertigo. If you or your child has these symptoms, see your doctor before trying any of the remedies in this chapter.

Weird & wacky

These cures should be labeled "weird, wacky, and disgusting." The first, mentioned in several compilations of old home remedies, calls for putting drops of urine in the affected ear. It's even been written that Elvis Presley's mother relied on this creepy remedy whenever The King had a childhood earache.

Another gross-sounding trick was to stuff the painful ear with a moist wad of chewing tobacco—or even to blow tobacco smoke into the ear. Thanks, but we'll pass on all of these. There's no known science to support any of them.

Garlic: the bacteria slayer

If you have garlic in the pantry, you might never need to give your child that pink prescription medicine ever again. Here's why: Garlic is Mother Nature's antibiotic. It contains compounds that kill bacteria and relieve inflammation. Some experts speculate that garlic combats bacteria differently than antibiotics. Since garlic doesn't rely on mimicking and interrupting the bacteria's defense mechanisms (like antibiotics do), bacteria don't fight against it. Thus, they don't mutate and become resistant to the cure.

Herbalists and doctors schooled in natural medicine say that using garlic oil in the ear eases ear pain because it migrates past the eardrum to alleviate the infection.

Here are five ways to harness garlic's power to clear up ear infections, including how to make garlic oil.

1. If your children get ear infections frequently, peel and finely chop garlic cloves from two or three bulbs. Place in a clean glass jar. Cover completely with olive oil and steep in the refrigerator for a week. At the end of the week, strain out the garlic and pour some oil into a little dropper bottle. To use, warm it slightly by standing the dropper bottle in a bowl of hot water. Add three or four drops to the affected ear and gently cover the opening with a cotton ball. Store the leftover oil in the refrigerator in a labeled and dated jar.

2. If you need garlic oil immediately, use a garlic crusher or mince the garlic as fine as you can and let it steep, covered in olive oil, for at least 15 minutes. Strain it and keep leftover oil in the refrigerator. Warm it slightly before dropping it into the affected ear with an ear dropper. Lightly cover the ear opening with a cotton ball.

3. Eat one or two raw cloves every day while you or your child is fighting the infection. One approach: Chop the fresh garlic, mix it with olive oil, and spread it on toast.

4. Mix chopped garlic with some warm honey and eat it right off the spoon. Never give honey to babies under 1 year old.

5. Squeeze a clove of garlic and put a few drops of the juice in the ear. Repeat three times a day.

fatigue

People complain of feeling drained and exhausted so often that doctors say fatigue is the leading reason for doctor's office visits. Often, simple measures can combat the problem. Sometimes the remedies may seem counterintuitive: Exercise, for example, is one of the best ways to beat fatigue. Sleeping too much, on the other hand, may not be helpful at all. But these quick kitchen pick-me-ups can be just what the doctor ordered.

first things first

Often, fatigue problems are nothing more than a symptom of bad sleeping habits. So start there. Are you getting seven to eight hours of sleep every night? If not, take these measures to remedy the situation:

• Establish a regular bed and wake time, and stick to it—even on the weekend.

• Likewise, establish a consistent "wind-down" bedtime routine, and give yourself enough time to complete it.

• As part of that wind-down period, turn off the television and the computer. But feel free to play relaxing music.

• Avoid nicotine, alcohol and caffeine close to bedtime. Any of these will disrupt your sleep.

• Increase your daytime activity level, including getting exercise. In addition to so many other health benefits, it helps to make you legitimately tired at night.

• Create a sleep-conducive environment that is dark, quiet, and comfortable.

Pantry
HEALERS

Apple cider vinegar

Bitters

Blackstrap molasses

Cranberry juice

Iron-rich foods

Lime juice

Peppermint essential oil

Rosemary essential oil

Tea

If your fatigue persists, even after you've taken steps to treat it, let your doctor know. When fatigue accompanies a sudden onset of abdominal pain, shortness of breath, or severe headache, seek immediate medical attention or call 911. Extreme exhaustion, alone or along with other symptoms, can signal a heart attack, especially for women. Other chronic symptoms that require a doctor's attention are muscle aches, nausea, depression, fever, or difficulty seeing.

kitchen cabinet cures

Drink something bitter. A traditional herbalists' cure for fatigue—which is still prescribed today by doctors in Germany—is to drink a tonic made of bitter herbs. The thinking was that because these herbs improve digestion, they might also enhance nourishment. Thus, if fatigue was due to nutritional deficits, a bitter tonic could turn things around. Whether or not that's true is debatable, but this modern take on an old-fashioned tonic is a real eye-opener—and there's a good chance you've got a bottle stashed along with your cocktail-making supplies. Shake several dashes of Angostura bitters into a tall glass of club soda or tonic water on ice. If nothing else, the sprightly taste will refresh and enliven you.

Spritz yourself awake. The scent of peppermint is known for its invigorating properties. Add 30 drops peppermint essential oil to water or witch hazel in a 4-ounce spray mister. Use freely to mist the air around you when you need some reawakening.

Or try this fragrant refresher. For a quick pick-me-up, put two drops of peppermint or rosemary essential oil on a tissue or handkerchief, hold it to your nose, and breathe deeply. If you have more time, try adding two drops of peppermint oil to cool bathwater along with four drops of rosemary oil for an invigorating soak.

Try tea and see. If you need a caffeinated pick-me-up, choose tea over coffee. One study found that drinking tea all day improved alertness and performance just as well as coffee and was less likely to disrupt sleep.

Have a cocktail. No, not a martini. Alcohol will only make you more fatigued. As a quick pick-me-up, try drinking a small glass of chilled cranberry juice with a splash of fresh lime juice.

Beat workout exhaustion. Exercise and sometimes extreme stress cause lactic acid to build up in the body, causing fatigue. Interestingly, the amino acids contained in apple cider vinegar act as an antidote. What's more, apple cider vinegar contains potassium and enzymes that may relieve that tired feeling. Next time you're feeling beat, add a tablespoon or two of apple cider vinegar to a glass of chilled vegetable drink or to a glass of water.

Drink something sweet. An old remedy for fatigue is molasses, probably on the theory that it contains iron, which could counter anemia. Try stirring 1 tablespoon blackstrap molasses into 1 cup of hot water next time fatigue catches up with you.

||||||||||||||||||||||||||||||||||||||||||||||||||||||||||||||||||||||||||||||||||||||||||||||||||||||||||||||||||||||||||||

There's an iron mine in your pantry

Iron deficiency is the most common cause of anemia, leading to a low volume of red blood cells in your body. Symptoms include weakness, pallor, fatigue, and brittle nails. If you suspect anemia, check with your doctor. Most cases are caused by blood loss (for example, from a bleeding ulcer or heavy menstrual flow).

The solution to anemia is right there in your pantry, where many iron-rich foods are stocked.

Aim for: The recommended amount of iron is 8 milligrams per day for men and menopausal women and 18 milligrams for menstruating women.

Helpful hint: Our bodies absorb iron much better from meat than from plant foods. If you get most of your iron from vegetarian sources like beans and peas, eat them with foods like citrus fruits that are high in vitamin C, which aids iron absorption.

Food	Standard Amount	Iron (mg)	Calories
Clams, canned, drained	3 oz.	23.8	126
Fortified ready-to-eat cereals (various)	about 1 oz.	1.8 –21.1	54–127
Fortified instant cooked cereals (various)	1 packet	4.9–8.1	Varies
Pumpkin and squash seed kernels, roasted	1 oz.	4.2	148
White beans, canned	½ cup	3.9	153
Blackstrap molasses	1 tablespoon	3.5	47
Lentils, cooked	½ cup	3.3	115
Kidney beans, cooked	½ cup	2.6	112
Sardines, canned in oil, drained	3 oz.	2.5	177
Chickpeas, cooked	½ cup	2.4	134
Prune juice	¾ cup	2.3	136
Shrimp, canned	3 oz.	2.3	102
Cowpeas, cooked	½ cup	2.2	100
Lima beans, cooked	½ cup	2.2	108
Soybeans, green, cooked	½ cup	2.2	127
Navy beans, cooked	½ cup	2.1	127
Refried beans	½ cup	2.1	118

fever

You're miserable when you have a fever. You're likely to feel boiling hot one minute, shivery cold the next. You're weak as a kitten and feel just plain awful all over. Bacterial or viral infections, such as tonsillitis or the flu, are usually the cause. Though it makes you feel miserable, a fever is actually part of your body's sophisticated immune system. You can make yourself feel better with these easy pantry fixes.

first things first

When you have a fever, the last thing you want to do is push through it by maintaining your usual schedule. Instead, follow this tried and true advice:

• Get into bed or onto your couch, and cover yourself up.
• Have hot tea and plenty of liquids at the ready.
• Settle in for a day or two of pure rest and relaxation.

kitchen cabinet cures

Bathe away a fever. To help bring down a high fever, take lukewarm or cool sponge baths once an hour or more frequently if necessary. Or just soak washcloths in cool water and apply them to your wrists, forehead, and neck. If you like, suck on ice chips spritzed with a little lemon juice to moisturize your mouth. Finally, drink water and other liquids liberally to prevent dehydration. Lukewarm

Pantry HEALERS

Cayenne

Chamomile tea

Cinnamon

Coriander

Cream of tartar

Ginger

Lavender
  essential oil

Lemon

Mustard powder

Peppermint
  essential oil

Rosemary

Rubbing alcohol

Thyme

Witch hazel

sponge baths cool the body slowly, and drinking liquids prevents dehydration.

Fight fire with spices. According to Ayurvedic healers who practice traditional Indian medicine, cinnamon, coriander, cayenne, and ginger promote sweating and can help break a fever. Use as much of the spicy stuff as you can comfortably stand. Add coriander, ginger, and cayenne freely to chicken broth to sip while you're recuperating. Sprinkle toast liberally with cinnamon or add it to tea.

Try a German fever cure. This is a popular concoction for lowering a fever, especially among folks of German descent. Add the juice of 1 lemon and 1 teaspoon cream of tartar to 16 ounces of hot water. Sweeten to taste with honey and sip slowly.

Work up a sweat with ginger tea. This fever remedy hails from all over the world—healers throughout North America, China, India, and the Middle East swear by it. Ginger contains anti-inflammatory compounds, some of which have mild aspirin-like effects. What's more, herbalists classify ginger as a diaphoretic, which means it makes you sweat, and sweating is a sure path to fever reduction. To make an effective fever tea, thinly slice a 2- to 3-inch-long piece of ginger and put it in a pot with a quart of water. Bring to a boil, then simmer over very low heat for 30 minutes, covered. Cool for another 30 minutes. Strain and drink a cup three times a day, sweetened with honey. No fresh ginger? Raid your spice rack for ginger powder. Add a teaspoon to a cup of boiled water, cover, and steep for 10 minutes. Strain before drinking. As with any remedy, check with your doctor before using if you're pregnant.

When to Call THE DOCTOR

If a fever lasts longer than three days, rises above 103°F, or is accompanied by a severe headache with stiff neck, a productive cough, abdominal pain, or painful urination, see a doctor. Also consult a doctor for fever in babies under six months old or in the elderly. Note that the body's temperature varies by as much as 2°F during the day, being lowest in the morning. Rectal temperature is usually about 1°F higher than other temperature measurements.

Caution: aspirin and children

Never give aspirin to a child with a fever, as it may increase the risk of a serious neurological illness called Reye's syndrome. Acetaminophen will bring the fever down safely. If a child has a temperature of 104°F or above, give acetaminophen and a sponge bath of lukewarm water. Continue sponge bathing until the temperature drops below 102°F. In adults as well as children, high fevers pose the risk of dehydration, so be sure to drink plenty of liquids.

Go soak your feet. A spicy foot bath can help ease fever by drawing blood to the feet. This eases the pressure on the blood vessels in your head and increases circulation. To a basin full of hot water, add a teaspoon of mustard powder. Stir well and soak your feet for 15 minutes or so. Wrap the rest of yourself up in a cuddly blanket.

 recipes for healing

Fragrant Fever Spritzer

Spraying pulse points with a cool, soothing solution feels great when you're hot and feverish. The pulse points are the places on the body where you can easily feel your heart rate when you touch them with your fingers—typically inside your wrists, just under each side of the jaw, and the back of the knees.

> ¼ cup rubbing alcohol
> ¼ cup witch hazel
> 3 drops peppermint essential oil
> 2 drops lavender essential oil

1. In a clean spray bottle, combine the rubbing alcohol, witch hazel, peppermint oil, and lavender oil. Shake to mix and then chill in the refrigerator.
2. Spray onto pulse points to reduce fever, avoiding eyes and mouth.

Coriander-Cinnamon Fever Chiller

This pungent tea contains spices with strong anti-fever properties.

> ½ teaspoon powdered coriander
> ½ teaspoon cinnamon
> ¼ teaspoon of powdered ginger

1. Add spices to cup of boiling water. Let it steep, covered, for 10 minutes, then drink.

Herb Tea Footbath

These herbs have a combination of powers that can help bring down a fever.

> 1 tablespoon dried peppermint
> 2 chamomile tea bags
> 1 tablespoon dried thyme
> 1 tablespoon dried rosemary

1. Bring the peppermint, chamomile tea bags, thyme, and rosemary to a boil in 2 quarts of water, then cover and simmer for 20 minutes. Allow the brew to cool till it is comfortably hot, then strain into a foot basin.
2. Wrap up in a blanket and immerse your feet in the tea for 15 to 20 minutes, during which time you should start sweating.

flatulence

You go to great lengths to avoid it. Teen comedies trumpet it. From Aristophanes to Chaucer to Mark Twain, great writers have satirized it. Since the dawn of human existence, for reasons that are unclear to folks of delicate sensibilities, public flatulence makes people laugh. Until it happens to you. At that point, it's just one great social faux pas you wish you could erase. Most healthy people pass gas several times a day, but excessive intestinal gas can point to a digestive disorder. It's an easy problem to remedy with these simple home remedies.

first things first

We all know that certain foods, like beans, are almost certain to fill up your gas tank. If that's a problem for you, try taking Beano, an over-the-counter supplement that counters the bean-gas effect.

kitchen cabinet cures

Spoon up some soda. To remedy a gassy digestive system, mix 1 teaspoon baking soda in a small glass of water, spritz in some lemon juice, and sip slowly.

Chew up a spoonful of seeds. Fennel seeds have a specific action that releases trapped intestinal gas. Simply chew up—thoroughly—a teaspoon or so of fennel seeds after a meal.

Pantry HEALERS

Baking soda
Brandy
Cayenne
Chamomile tea
Crystallized ginger
Cumin
Epazote
Fennel seeds
Marjoram
Peppermint tea
Turmeric

When to Call
THE DOCTOR

Rarely does flatulence signal a medical problem. If you're frequently plagued, try changing your diet to avoid gas-producing foods, such as beans and lentils and dairy products containing lactose. If your problem is associated with vomiting, diarrhea, constipation, heartburn, or unexplained weight loss, see your doctor for a checkup. He or she may want to examine you for other indications of the condition known as irritable bowel syndrome or other ailments. Also, severe flatulence that doesn't go away can sometimes be a symptom of gallbladder problems, an inflammatory condition in the intestines, or colon cancer.

Brew some mint tea. Peppermint tea is such a gentle and time-honored treatment for flatulence that hospitals often give it to new mothers following Caesarean section births. Simply steep a peppermint tea bag in just-boiled water, covered, for 10 minutes, and sip slowly after eating.

Seek spicy antidotes. For some gas-producing foods, there's a corresponding anti-gas spice. Take beans, for example. Adding a teaspoon or so of ground cumin not only perks up their flavor, but it will counteract their propensity to produce flatulence. Other anti-gas pairings include chopping crystallized ginger into ice cream (it complements most flavors) or sprinkling cayenne onto cheeses. The leafy Mexican herb epazote has a long-held reputation for "de-gassing" foods. Add some to your chili or stew.

Try turmeric for relief. Ayurvedic healers swear by turmeric as a quick source of gas relief. Boil a teaspoon of turmeric in a cup of water. Strain and drink immediately.

Tap into the liquor pantry. Many home remedy experts say that a little brandy after a meal will help with digestion and reduce gassiness. Either take a teaspoon straight, or add 2 teaspoons to a cup of water and drink.

 recipe for healing

Anti-gas Tea

Herbalists call these herbs "carminative," which means they help dispel gas, aid digestion, and ease intestinal spasms. This makes enough tea to take in a thermos and sip all day long.

> 4 chamomile tea bags
> 4 peppermint tea bags
> 1 teaspoon crushed fennel seeds
> 1 teaspoon dried marjoram

Steep tea bags, fennel seeds, and marjoram in 1 quart boiling water, covered, for 10 minutes. Strain. Chill and drink it cold or keep it hot in a thermos.

foot problems

So many things can make your dogs ache that it's hard to know where to begin. Shoes that don't fit properly or that force your feet into impossible angles are a good place to start. Running, jogging, or performing other athletics in shoes that don't offer proper support also make the list. Beyond foot pain are these discomforts: feet that feel perpetually chilly and ingrown toenails. You'll find answers to all these minor woes right behind your pantry door.

first things first

In most cases, healthy feet are directly related to right-sized shoes:

• Have your feet measured properly at a good shoe store. Measure width as well as length. You might be surprised to learn that you've been scrunching your feet into the wrong-sized shoes for years.

• Find out from your doctor whether you have flat feet or fallen arches. Or merely show your worn shoes to a good shoe salesperson; they can often tell from the wear pattern whether you have either. Some podiatrists and chiropractors now use a special gizmo that you step on, and it instantly assesses any problems.

• If you learn that your feet need more support, consider getting special shoe inserts (called orthotics) from your podiatrist or medical supply store.

Pantry HEALERS

Apple cider vinegar
Cayenne
Cinnamon
Olive oil
Peppermint tea
Thyme

kitchen cabinet cures

Give tootsies a vigorous rub. To stimulate circulation and relieve pain, massage your feet (better yet, get your loving partner to do it for you) in equal quantities of olive oil and apple cider vinegar.

Try some hydrotherapy. You'll love this one because it makes your feet feel like new. Fill one basin with cold water and another with water as hot as you can comfortably stand. Sit in a comfortable chair, and place your feet in the cold water. After 5 minutes, switch to the hot water. Repeat. This "hydromassage" alternately dilates and constricts blood vessels in your feet, boosting circulation.

Soak in thyme tea. In a just-released study, researchers discovered that thyme contains the same kind of COX-II inhibitors as nonsteroidal anti-inflammatory drugs, such as ibuprofen. Make a strong tea with 2 tablespoons of dried thyme in a quart of boiling water. Cover the pot and simmer for 20 minutes. Let it cool until it's hot enough for you to comfortably stand the temperature. Then soak your feet in the tea for 15 to 20 minutes.

Minty foot energizer. After hours of standing all day, especially during the summer, refresh your aching feet with this tea: Add three or four peppermint tea bags to a quart or two of just-boiled water, let steep for 15 minutes, and cool the tea. Pour it in a foot basin or a foot spa, add some ice cubes, and soak for 15 minutes or so.

Spice up cold feet. If you're going to be outdoors on a frigid winter day, try this warmer-upper. Sprinkle a little ground red pepper (cayenne) into your socks. The stimulating heat will keep tootsies warm. Tote a clean pair of socks with you in case you find the cayenne irritating.

Have a glass of cinnamon. Chinese healers say that drinking a little cinnamon water will stimulate circulation and keep feet (and hands) warm. Just mix a half-teaspoon into a glass of hot water. Let it steep for a few minutes and drink three times a day. Bonus: Cinnamon also helps lower blood sugar and cholesterol.

When to Call THE DOCTOR

Don't worry if your feet hurt occasionally. But be sure to visit a podiatrist if walking first thing in the morning is difficult or if the painful area is swollen or discolored. You may have a broken bone, an inflamed tendon, or a pinched nerve. And see the doctor if you regularly have pain after walking long distances or working out on treadmills or elliptical machines—this could indicate flat feet or other structural problems. A painful, burning sensation in the feet might mean you have diabetes or thyroid disease. If you have diabetes, see your doctor at once if a cut, sore, bruise, or blister on your foot doesn't start to heal after one day.

gum problems

Spend a few minutes each day being compulsive about your oral hygiene, and you'll stand a good chance of warding off gum problems, including gingivitis and periodontal disease. Deal with plaque by visiting your dentist at least twice a year, and invest extra time in brushing (use a soft-bristled brush and pay special attention to your gum line) and flossing your teeth. You can also keep your gums nice and healthy with some easy pantry treatments.

first things first

Mouth-cleaning gear keeps getting fancier and more high-tech, but the fundamentals haven't changed:

• Brush your teeth and gums every morning and evening, and even better, after every meal.

• Use floss or interdental brushes between the teeth at least once a day.

• Use an antibacterial mouthwash containing tea tree or myrrh.

• Avoid smoking.

• Don't chew on toothpicks or other hard objects.

• See your dentist for cleanings at least twice a year. Most gingivitis will resolve quickly and easily if the plaque is removed from around the necks of the teeth.

Pantry HEALERS

Aloe

Antibacterial mouthwash

Black tea

Chamomile tea

Echinacea

Green tea

Hydrogen peroxide

Myrrh essential oil

Orange pekoe tea

Salt

Sesame seeds

Sunflower seeds

Thyme

Witch hazel

kitchen cabinet cures

Massage gums with aloe. Aloe helps damaged tissue heal and soothes irritation, which makes it a perfect treatment for sore gums. Scrape a few spoonfuls of aloe gel from a cut stalk into a saucer. Dip a soft-bristled toothbrush into the aloe and gently massage the gums by stroking the brush over them in a back and forth motion. Dip the brush in the aloe every time you move to a new spot. Work your way bit by bit until you've covered the entire surface of your gums. This helps stimulate blood circulation and heals the tissue.

Swish some salt. To sooth gum pain and reduce swelling, swish your mouth for 30 seconds or so with salt water (1 teaspoon salt mixed into a glass of warm water). Or mix hydrogen peroxide 50:50 with warm water and swish through your mouth for 30 seconds or so.

Gnaw on sesame seeds. Both sesame seeds and sunflower seeds contain minerals that contribute to healthy teeth and gums. Chew a spoonful slowly every day to help strengthen gum tissue.

Use a cold herb to treat gums. That bottle of echinacea you use to head off colds comes in mighty handy as a treatment for sore gums. It promotes healing, and it acts as a local anesthetic to relieve pain. You can apply liquid echinacea directly to sore gums with a cotton swab, or you

Treat your teeth, protect your heart

Here's a health flash you don't want to miss: People with chronic bacterial infections of the gums are nearly twice as likely to have fatal heart attacks as those with healthy gums. That's right. Brushing and flossing your teeth don't just brighten your smile—they can also save your life.

In a University of Minnesota study of more than 700 men and women with no history of heart disease, researchers found a direct link between missing teeth (an indicator of serious dental disease) and plaque buildup in the arteries. Other studies have linked periodontal

(gum) disease with increased resting heart rate, abnormal electrocardiograms, and poor blood sugar control—all symptoms of or contributors to heart disease.

University of Michigan researchers who studied 320 U.S. veterans went so far as to conclude that dental disease was a larger risk factor for heart disease than being overweight, having high cholesterol, not exercising, or smoking. So run, don't walk, to the phone, and make that dental appointment right now.

can add a teaspoon of echinacea tincture to a half cup of warm water and swish vigorously through your gums for at least a minute. Repeat daily.

Make an herbal mouthwash. Add 1 teaspoon dried thyme to a cup of just-boiled water. Thyme contains compounds that relieve pain and kill bacteria. Steep, covered, for 15 minutes before straining. Cool and use as a mouthwash two or three times a day.

Press on some orange pekoe. Tea contains astringent tannic acid that shrinks swollen tissues and helps staunch bleeding. If bleeding and inflammation persist, fold the bag in half and bite down on it.

Calm gums with chamomile. Studies have shown that using chamomile tea as a mouthwash reduces gum pain and helps heal gingivitis. Just pour a cup of hot water over two chamomile tea bags, cover, steep for 10 minutes, and cool to room temperature. Remove the tea bags, take a mouthful of tea and swish it around vigorously for several minutes before spitting out. Repeat until you've used the entire cup. Do this daily for best results. You can also press the wet tea bags for a minute or two against any areas that are particularly irritated.

 recipe for healing

Super Healing Mouth Rinse

Black tea and witch hazel are rich in tannins, which improve tissue tone. Green tea is an antioxidant and lessens inflammation, and myrrh is a time-honored treatment for gum problems.

> 2 black tea bags
> 2 green tea bags
> ¾ cup boiling water
> 1 tablespoon witch hazel
> 5 drops myrrh essential oil (optional)

1. Place black and green teas in a bowl and cover with boiling water. Cover bowl and steep for 30 minutes. Strain.
2. Add the witch hazel and myrrh oil. Mix well. Store in a dark glass bottle.
3. To use, shake well and swish 1 to 2 tablespoons around the mouth. Do not swallow. Store in a cool place. Use within one week.

headache

Pantry HEALERS

Butterbur

Chamomile tea

Cloves

Fennel seeds

Gingerroot

Lavender
essential oil

Magnesium
supplements

Olive oil

Pain reliever
(acetaminophen,
aspirin, ibuprofen,
naproxen)

Peppermint
essential oil

Rosemary

Rosemary
essential oil

Thyme

Thyme essential oil

Vitamin B$_2$

So many things can make your head ache. Deadlines. Arguments. Irksome bosses. Traffic jams. Even good things can give you a pain in the head—on the Mayo Clinic Web site, "ice cream headaches" has its own category (many of us know it as "brain freeze"). Generally speaking, headaches are your body's response to physical or emotional stress. That stress can make the muscles in your head and neck contract to create tension headaches. Or it can make blood vessels constrict and later expand to produce migraines or vascular headaches. And if your sinuses are congested or infected, pounding headaches often result. Despite the discomfort, most headaches are temporary and respond quite nicely to do-it-yourself pantry treatments.

first things first

Sometimes the obvious solutions *are* the best solutions. When a simple, run-of-the-mill headache starts coming on, do these two things:

• Immediately take an over-the-counter pain reliever, such as acetaminophen, aspirin, ibuprofen, or naproxen, as directed on the bottle.

• Distance yourself from whatever triggered the headache, be it a stressful situation, bright sunlight, or loud music. If you can, get to a quiet, calm room with dim light and relax for 15 minutes.

kitchen cabinet cures

Soothe on fragrant oil. To relieve headache pain, dab a drop or two of thyme or rosemary essential oil on each temple and on your forehead. Rub gently into the skin, then sit quietly for several minutes. In a 2010 study, researchers discovered that thyme and rosemary oils contain carvacrol, a substance that acts as a COX-II inhibitor, much like non-steroidal anti-inflammatory drugs, such as ibuprofen, do.

Enjoy some ginger tea. Ginger may work against migraines by inhibiting prostaglandin synthesis. What's more, ginger helps quell the nausea that often accompanies migraines. Make a tea by gently simmering three quarter-sized slices of gingerroot in 2 cups of water, covered, for 30 minutes.

Pain-easing sweet tea. Taking a break in your busy schedule can relieve some of the tension that causes many headaches. Chamomile tea has compounds that help ease pain and relax you. Brew up a cup using one chamomile tea bag to a cup of just-boiled water. Allow to steep, covered, for 10 minutes. Sweeten with honey, if desired. Take a few minutes to sip the hot tea slowly while sitting in a quiet spot.

Have an herbal footbath. Some natural healers believe footbaths are powerful remedies for headaches. The hot water draws blood to your feet, easing the pressure on the blood vessels in your head. When a few drops of peppermint and/or lavender essential oils are added, the aroma provides soothing relief.

Mine some magnesium. Headache researchers say that migraine sufferers should keep this essential mineral in their medicine chests. Turns out, migraineurs (the term docs use to describe folks who get these head-splitters) have low levels of magnesium in their brains during attacks and may also have a general magnesium deficiency. In fact, two placebo-controlled clinical studies have shown that taking magnesium supplements can prevent the headaches. Experts recommend taking 400 milligrams a day of chelated magnesium, magnesium oxide, or slow-release magnesium, all of which are available over the counter at your local drugstore. Note: Magnesium may cause diarrhea in some people.

When to Call THE DOCTOR

Most headaches are easily dealt with on your own and are of no medical concern. But if your headache is accompanied by any of these symptoms, see a doctor immediately. It could be a symptom of a much more serious condition.

- Sudden awakenings from sleep
- Blurry vision
- Confusion or slurred speech, especially after a blow to the head
- Difficulty moving any one part of your body
- Fever and a stiff neck
- Nausea
- Pain in or around your eyes
- Pain that is sudden and more severe than your typical headache

Take vitamin B₂. In one study, taking 400 milligrams of this vitamin, known as riboflavin, daily for three months slashed migraines by 50 percent in 59 percent of the volunteers, as opposed to just 15 percent in volunteers who took a placebo.

Go herbal on migraines. An herb called butterbur has proved itself so effective for migraine relief that physicians who specialize in treating migraines often recommend it. At least three studies have been conducted on Petadolex, an over-the-counter butterbur extract, and in each study, the herb has significantly reduced migraine attacks when compared to a placebo. Recommended dosage is 75 milligrams twice a day for one month, then 50 milligrams twice a day.

 recipes for healing

Pain-Relieving Compress

These herbs all contain carvacrol, a compound that suppresses the COX-II enzyme—which means they have the same action as ibuprofen and other nonsteroidal anti-inflammatory drugs.

> I tablespoon dried thyme
> I tablespoon dried rosemary
> I teaspoon cloves, crushed
> I teaspoon fennel seeds, crushed

1. Add the thyme, rosemary, cloves, and fennel seeds to 3 cups of water in a pot. Bring to a boil, then simmer gently, covered, for 30 minutes. Let cool till it's comfortably warm.

2. Soak a cotton cloth in the brew and wring out excess liquid.

3. Place the compress on your forehead or the back of your neck to relax the tight muscles that are often the cause of a tension headache. You can also chill the brew and make a cold compress. This will constrict the blood vessels and reduce blood flow, which may relieve a vascular headache.

Headache Rub

The combination of fragrant aroma and gentle massage can quiet a painful headache.

> 10 drops olive oil
> 3 drops peppermint essential oil
> 3 drops lavender essential oil

1. In a small bowl, mix the olive oil and the essential oils.

2. Dip your fingers into the oil and then massage the oil into the temples, along the hairline and the base of the skull, being careful not to get the oil in your eyes.

3. Wash your hands thoroughly after each application.

hemorrhoids

Topping the list of infernally irritating problems is hemorrhoids. Making matters worse, it's an intimate condition that most folks find too embarrassing to discuss—even with their doctors. These swollen varicose veins that appear in or around the anus have a variety of causes. Constipation (common during pregnancy) and dry stools rank high on the list. Also to blame are prolonged sitting or standing. Straining to pass hard, dry stools is a culprit, as is catching up on your reading while sitting on the "throne." A fiber-poor diet is a major contributor to the problem. The good news is, many pantry remedies are remarkably effective and may help you avoid more invasive medical treatments.

first things first
You can ease or even prevent hemorrhoids by losing weight, increasing water and fiber intake, and enjoying dried figs, prunes, and dates, which all have laxative properties. Other easy tips include:

• Wear cotton undies.

• Use plain white fragrance-free toilet tissue.

• Don't scratch itchy hemorrhoids.

• Take a warm sitz bath for 10 to 15 minutes twice a day.

• Limit the amount of time you sit on the john (forgo reading while you sit).

• Don't strain to move bowels.

• Cleanse with flushable, moistened wipes after each bowel movement.

Pantry
HEALERS

Aloe
Apple cider vinegar
Black tea
Chamomile tea
Epsom salts
Lavender
  essential oil
Witch hazel

It's risky to self-diagnose hemorrhoids. You can't really see what's going on, and the hemorrhoid can be symptomatic of something more serious. That's why doctors prefer you make an appointment rather than assuming you can figure out the problem and solution on your own. Severe pain can be a sign of a thrombosed hemorrhoid, which occurs when a vein ruptures or a blood clot occurs in the hemorrhoid. If these are treated within 24 hours, the blood clot can be removed with a local anesthetic. Rectal bleeding may be a hemorrhoid symptom, or it can signal something more serious, such as colon cancer.

kitchen cabinet cures

Try witch power. Witch hazel is a natural anti-inflammatory that shrinks swollen veins and can bring immediate relief. Chill the bottle for 15 minutes in the refrigerator, then soak a wad of cotton in it and place the cotton ball on the hemorrhoid. At night, tuck a soaked cotton ball against the area and put on cotton undies. You'll find it helps relieve pain and itching so you can sleep.

Dab on some vinegar. Apple cider vinegar helps bring down the swelling and eases inflamed hemorrhoids. Apply to a cotton ball and wipe across the anal area. If it stings or burns, dilute the vinegar 50-50 with water.

Smear on some aloe. Soothing, healing aloe gel is an ideal hemorrhoid healer. Just slash open a stalk and dip a gauze pad into the gel, then apply.

Bag the pain. Place a warm, wet black tea bag directly on those painful swellings. You can do it while sitting on the toilet. The warmth is soothing, and you get added benefit from one of tea's main components, tannic acid. It helps reduce swelling, and its astringent action helps stop the bleeding. You can also use a wet chamomile tea bag, which will lessen the inflammation.

Take an Epsom soak. Sit in a tub of warm water in which you've dissolved a cup or so of Epsom salts. The warm water eases pain, and the salts constrict the hemorrhoid. Do not try this if hemorrhoids are bleeding.

 ## recipe for healing

DIY Hemorrhoid Pads

These soothing, cooling pads work just as well as store-bought—and smell heavenly.

> ¼ cup witch hazel
> 10 drops lavender essential oil
> 2 tablespoons aloe vera gel, scraped from inside a fresh aloe leaf

1. In a shallow, open-mouthed jar with a tight-fitting lid, combine the witch hazel, lavender oil, and aloe vera gel. Saturate cotton gauze pads in the liquid and refrigerate for at least an hour.

2. Use a pad on the affected area when it burns and after each bowel movement. Store in the refrigerator for several days.

hiccups

There's something silly about having hiccups. Invariably, they make anyone within earshot giggle at you. But they probably weren't such a laugh riot for poor Charles Osborne from Anthon, Iowa, who hiccuped continuously from 1922 to 1990—producing an estimated 430 million hiccups over 68 years! Fortunately, most attacks are far more fleeting. In a nutshell, a hiccup is just an involuntary contraction of the diaphragm. This makes you suddenly draw in a breath, which is checked by the abrupt closing of the glottis (the space between the vocal cords). The result is the characteristic hiccup sound. Hiccups are usually harmless. If there's no one around to scare the wits out of you, try some of these simple tricks to make them go away.

first things first

As soon as hiccups start, drink some water and take some deep breaths. Often, that's enough to stymie an attack. If they continue, try some of our proven home remedies.

kitchen cabinet cures

Swallow something sweet. A spoonful of sugar is popular because its graininess could slightly irritate the esophagus, causing the phrenic nerves to "reset" themselves, although there is no proof of this.

... Or something sour. Take a teaspoonful of vinegar. Its sour taste could stop a hiccup in its tracks.

Pantry HEALERS

Chocolate (powdered drink mix)

Dill seeds

Honey

Hot sauce

Paper bag

Paper towel

Peanut butter

Sugar

Vinegar

Water

Weird
& wacky

We actually like this oddball remedy we discovered. It's just silly and distracting enough to make you forget to hiccup: Hold a penny between two toes and transfer it to two toes on your other foot. Don't let the penny touch the floor.

Sip some hot sauce. This probably works because the heat and burn are distracting enough to turn your body's focus on the burn, instead of the hiccup process.

Brown bag 'em. Breathe slowly and deeply into a small paper bag. (Stop if you feel light-headed.) This increases the carbon dioxide level in the blood and makes the diaphragm contract more deeply to bring in more oxygen, which may stop the spasms.

Chew up some dill. Here's a simple, pleasant-tasting trick: Slowly chew a teaspoon of dill seeds. This traditional cure may work because swallowing the seeds stimulates the vagus nerve to make the hiccups stop.

Try the paper towel trick. Place a single layer of paper towel over the top of a glass, then drink through the towel. You'll have to "pull" harder with your diaphragm to suck up the water, and concentrated gulping counteracts spasmodic muscle movements.

Enjoy a little honey. Put 1 teaspoon of honey, stirred in warm water, on the back of your tongue, and swallow it. Like dill, honey could potentially tickle the vagus nerve to make the hiccups stop.

Have some PB. A classic hiccups remedy involves eating a big spoonful of peanut butter. In the process of chewing and getting it off your tongue and teeth, your swallowing and breathing patterns are interrupted. And hence, the hiccups will be history.

Yummy chocolate remedy. Eat some powdered chocolate drink mix (cocoa or Ovaltine) right off the spoon. Swallowing the spoonful isn't easy and should short-circuit the hiccups.

Try the love cure

It's not scientifically proven, but this hiccup remedy that hails from North Carolina is sweet indeed: While you're hiccuping, focus on the person you love best. This bit of folklore goes on to state that if your beloved loves you back, your hiccups will cease.

indigestion

The term "indigestion" means different things to different people, and the territory of troubles it covers is huge. Just to clear up any confusion, indigestion and heartburn are two different problems. Heartburn produces a painful or burning sensation in the center of your chest, due to acid spilling upward into your esophagus. Indigestion happens further south: It produces bloating, a feeling of uncomfortable fullness during or after a meal, or pain or burning concentrated in the upper abdomen. Smokers, pregnant women, and people who are overweight are especially susceptible. Luckily, indigestion symptoms are especially easy to tame by employing simple lifestyle tweaks and easy home remedies.

first things first

These simple suggestions can help make bouts of indigestion a thing of the past:

• Eat smaller, more frequent meals.

• Avoid your triggers. Spicy or fatty foods, carbonated drinks, and alcohol are frequent tummy troublers.

• Don't smoke.

• Maintain a healthy weight.

• Take your time when you dine.

• Be active—exercise improves digestion.

Pantry HEALERS

Anise seeds

Apple cider vinegar

Baking soda

Bitter beer

Candied ginger

Caraway seeds

Chamomile tea

Dill seeds

Fennel seeds

Honey

Lemon

Mint tea

The vast majority of indigestion cases are simple, one-time affairs, easily cured with home remedies. But call 911 if you experience nausea along with sweating or an ache or pain in the chest; you may be having a heart attack. See your doctor if you have intense abdominal pain, especially if you also have black or bloody stools or if you're vomiting. And you need a checkup if indigestion lingers for more than a couple of weeks, despite your best attempts at self-care.

Weird & wacky

It's no surprise to us that a condition so ubiquitous would rack up scores and scores of crazy treatments. But these three tickled our funny bones:

• Bend over, turn over a rock, and walk forward without looking back.

• For a child's indigestion: Pass him backward around a table leg seven times.

• Execute a somersault.

kitchen cabinet cures

Make a four-seed chew. Mix a batch of this seedy chew, which combats indigestion by helping your system expel excess gas. Take 1 teaspoon each of fennel, dill, anise, and caraway seeds and blend. Chew up a half-teaspoon or so, slowly, when you're having indigestion after you've eaten a big, spicy, or fatty meal. You might see this same mix in Indian restaurants, where it is often put in bowls for customers to sample as they leave.

Order up some mint or chamomile. A steaming cup of one of these teas will quickly dispel that dyspeptic feeling. Simply use one of either kind of tea bag to a cup of water. Cover and steep for 10 minutes before drinking. Many restaurants stock these two calming brews, so have it after dinner if you've eaten something rich that might not agree with you.

Sip this before eating. If you know you're going to indulge in foods that will make you sorry later, try this folk remedy first. Add 1 teaspoon of honey and 1 teaspoon apple cider vinegar to a glass of warm water and drink it 30 minutes before you dine.

Soda to the rescue. Stir a teaspoon of baking soda into a glass of water, add a few drops of lemon juice, and drink it. If your stomach is too acidic, this solution neutralizes stomach acid and helps relieve painful gas. In very rare cases, baking soda has been known to explode in the stomach and cause tearing, so squirt the lemon juice into the water first, to dispel some of the gas before it hits your stomach.

Nibble on candy. Candied ginger, that is. Ginger slices that have been dried and sugared are sold in supermarkets and health or natural food stores. They keep forever in the pantry and taste yummy. Two or three pieces can tame your tummy woes. This makes a great remedy for children's minor stomach aches.

Have half a bitter beer. Beers that have a bitter bite are rich in hops, an herb that helps stimulate digestion. But don't get carried away—more than a half glass of beer will depress your digestion.

insomnia

If you listen to the chatter around the office coffee machine every morning, you'd think that tossing and turning is our national pastime. So few people admit to getting a good night's sleep these days that everyone seems to have an opinion on the subject. The reasons we sleep so poorly are many: the stresses of 21st-century living, multitasking, financial and family concerns, health problems, bedrooms loaded with blinking, high-tech electronics...the list goes on and on. Take comfort from knowing that, as with any other health issue, admitting that you have a problem puts you on the path to solving it. These easily made home remedies will help improve your sleep.

first things first

One of the first pieces of advice you'd be likely to hear from a sleep medicine specialist is to "improve your sleep hygiene." Interpretation: Sleeping poorly can often be traced to having bad habits that can be easily fixed. Here, from the National Sleep Foundation, are some tips to help you have good hygiene of the sleep variety:

• Establish a regular bed and wake time.

• Avoid nicotine altogether and avoid caffeine close to bedtime.

• Avoid alcohol in the hours approaching sleep time.

• Exercise regularly (but complete your workout at least three hours before bedtime).

Pantry HEALERS

Chamomile tea

Lavender essential oil

Mandarin oranges

Milk

Pumpkin seeds

Sesame seeds

Sugar

Sunflower seeds

Tarragon

There's certainly no science for this nutty-sounding folk remedy, but who knows? Maybe onion vapors contain a sleep-inducing substance that researchers have yet to discover. We'd consider trying this one only as a last resort. Cut up a yellow onion and put it into a canning jar. Screw on the cover and put the jar on your nightstand. If you have trouble falling asleep, or wake up in the middle of the night, open the jar and take a few deep breaths. Then close the jar, lie back, and visualize calming images. With any luck, the next time you open your eyes it will be morning.

• Establish a consistent relaxing "wind-down" bedtime routine.

• Create a sleep-conducive environment that is dark, quiet, and comfortable.

• Discuss the appropriate way to take any sleep aid with a health care professional.

kitchen cabinet cures

Brew this herbal nightcap. Sip a strong cup of chamomile tea (made with two tea bags) before going to bed every night. When sleep comes more easily, cut back to using one tea bag (continued use of the stronger concentration can cause sleeplessness to return).

Make lavender oil your friend. In at least one study, inhaling lavender essential oil before bedtime helped people with insomnia sleep better. You can use the sweetly scented oil in several ways:

• Massage a few drops of lavender essential oil into your temples before going to bed.

• Sprinkle a few drops of oil onto your pillowcase each night (it won't stain).

• Use an aromatherapy diffuser to waft the scent throughout your bedroom.

• Take a relaxing hot bath before bedtime. Add lavender essential oil or lavender bath salts to the tub. Light some lavender candles and play relaxing music, then dry off and slip into bed.

Lavender essential oil is widely available at health and natural food stores. Make sure to buy 100 percent pure essential oil, rather than a cheaper perfumed oil product.

Go on, count those sheep

Believe it or not, there's something to the age-old ritual of counting sheep. Picturing the woolly livestock engages the right side of the brain, while counting them uses the left, effectively preventing you from concentrating on anything else: work problems, worries, or the fear of not falling asleep.

Nosh on some seeds. Pumpkin, sesame, and sunflower seeds all contain L-tryptophan, a substance the body uses to convert to the calming neurotransmitter serotonin. Try nibbling on a handful of seeds nightly 30 minutes before bedtime.

Sleep like royalty. If you're a terrible sleeper, you owe it to yourself to make an investment in the most comfortable bedding you can afford. Look for 100 percent cotton sheets with a thread count of 250 or higher for the most softness. If you've been sleeping on the same mattress for more than five years, consider getting a new one—and take your time picking one out. And change your pillows: Some people find that "memory foam" pillows can make sleeping more comfortable.

Try a fruity dessert. Canned mandarin oranges are mentioned in folk medicine as having sleep-inducing properties. There's no science to back this remedy, so it's on the list of otherwise healthy remedies that certainly can't hurt and might just help the situation. Choose brands canned in their natural juice rather than heavy sugar syrups.

Go from pancakes to pillows. Buckwheat pillows are stuffed with the well-cleaned hulls of a buckwheat stalk. Users swear by their comfort. In one study of customer satisfaction of 10 pillow types, buckwheat came in second. Originally from Japan, buckwheat pillows are becoming available worldwide as healthy, ultra-comfortable alternatives to foam or feather pillows.

Try tarragon. A traditional French home remedy for insomnia is to make a tea from dried tarragon. Put about 2 teaspoons of the herb into 2 cups of boiling water, cover, and let steep for about 30 minutes. Strain, then have a cup shortly before going to bed.

Make a milk cocktail. One of the best-known home remedies for insomnia is warm milk. But few know that having some carbs at the same time helps get the milk's tryptophan—the key amino acid for inducing sleep—to enter the brain. So folk healers say to heat the milk to just before boiling, then stir in a teaspoon of white or brown sugar. Consider adding a teaspoon of vanilla and a sprinkle of cinnamon on top, both for flavor and your health.

When to Call THE DOCTOR

If you've tried the remedies in this chapter and nothing helps you sleep, see your doctor for a checkup if insomnia persists. Many conditions and some medications have sleeplessness as a symptom. After ruling out physical problems, your doctor may refer you to a sleep clinic for treatment.

laryngitis

You're croaking instead of speaking—that is, if you can make any noise at all. Chances are, you've either got a bad sore throat, which has swollen your vocal chords, or you've been overusing your voice (think politicians on election night). The result is laryngitis, an inflammation of the larynx (voice box), the part of the windpipe that houses your vocal cords. Normally, the vocal cords open and shut when you speak. When the vocal cords swell, they vibrate differently, which causes hoarseness. Smoking, allergies, sinus infections, dust, fumes, or even heartburn or bronchitis can cause a froggy voice. Key to home treatment is soothing the irritation, and that's easily done with ingredients you're likely to have on hand.

first things first

In addition to home remedies to soothe your vocal cords, do these for quick relief:

• Give your voice a rest and do your best not to talk until you're well on the way to healing.

• Don't whisper, either—it dries out your vocal chords.

• Whatever you do, don't smoke.

• Try not to "clear your voice."

• Don't drink alcohol.

• Use a humidifier or take herbal steams.

• Keep your throat moist by sucking on lozenges.

• Gargle several times a day with ½ teaspoon salt in a glass of warm water.

kitchen cabinet cures

Get some myrrh tincture. Unless the Wise Men visited you recently, you probably don't have this remedy in your medicine chest. But maybe you should: Herbalists consider myrrh the go-to treatment for healing oral problems. It kills pain and germs on contact and quickly combats inflammation. You can find myrrh tincture at health food stores—a little bottle lasts a long time. To treat laryngitis, add 30 drops to a glass of warm water and gargle six times a day. Don't use without diluting, and don't swallow it. Also, avoid if you're pregnant or nursing.

Have some sage-honey tea. Sage is said to help restore the voice, and honey is soothing and antiseptic. Use 1 teaspoon of dried sage to 1 cup of boiling water, cover and steep for 10 minutes, then strain. Sweeten with a couple of spoonfuls of honey and drink.

Spoon up a bowl of hot soup. Warm liquids, such as chicken broth, can help ease the discomfort. But spicy hot liquids help even more. Spike your soup with a sprinkle of cayenne or a few dashes of hot pepper sauce.

Sip some onion juice. Onions are a folk medicine staple. Like garlic, they're rich in compounds that quell inflammation and combat germs. An old home remedy for laryngitis is to drink a mixture of 2 teaspoons onion juice followed by a "chaser" of 1 teaspoon honey. Take those 3 teaspoonfuls every three hours. To get onion juice, press an onion half between two cutting boards and collect the juice that runs out. Of course, if you own a juicer, you don't have to use all that elbow grease.

Grab some gum before takeoff. When you travel by plane, chew gum or suck on lozenges. The cabin air is excessively dry, and your vocal cords suffer. If you keep your mouth closed and increase saliva production, you help prevent dehydration. And make it a point to down a glass of water each hour you're in flight.

When to Call THE DOCTOR

Usually laryngitis isn't serious, and you'll have your voice back in a few days. But if you're still hoarse after four or five days or if you're running a fever, let your doctor know. Persistent, unexplained hoarseness could signal something serious, especially if you're a smoker or tobacco chewer. See a doctor immediately or call 911 if your laryngitis is accompanied by pain so severe that you have trouble swallowing or if you're coughing up blood or wheezing.

Weird & wacky

For reasons we couldn't fathom, chestnut shells turn up in folklore as a laryngitis remedy. The directive is to chew the shells as if you were chewing gum. Frankly, we thought this treatment was just plain nutty until we came across a 2007 medical study—it suggested that the shells are actually loaded with antioxidants.

memory problems

Pantry HEALERS

Blueberry juice

Canned fish (salmon, sardines, herring, mackerel)

Cinnamon

Flaxseeds

Green tea

Prunes

Pumpkin seeds

Raisins

Sage tea

Sesame seeds

Shiitake mushrooms

Spinach

Sunflower seeds

Turmeric

Most middle-aged folks can lay claim to at least a few of these so-called "senior moments" in which our memory seems to fail us. As we age, our brains store information differently, making it harder for us to recall facts. But aging isn't always the problem. Simply trying to juggle too many important details can wreak havoc on your focus. Thyroid disorders can affect memory, as can medications, including those for high blood pressure, anxiety, and cancer. Believe it or not, you can often rescue a less-than-perfect memory with simple pantry cures.

first things first

Feeling forgetful lately? Take a close look at how much sleep you've been getting. Chronic sleep deprivation can shrink the hippocampus, the region of the brain responsible for accurate memory. In fact, studies have shown that just a few days of insufficient sleep time stresses the brain and could potentially mess up your memory. Other memory-slayers include smoking (even secondhand smoke can affect memory) as well as abusing alcohol and recreational drugs.

kitchen cabinet cures

Become a seed freak. Brain experts recommend nibbling on seeds to help protect your memory. That's because seeds—especially flax, sunflower, sesame, and pumpkin—are rich in magnesium, a mineral that helps protect brain cells from overstimulation, which is deadly to cells. What's more, seeds are laced with brain-healthy omega-3 fatty acids that help keep cell membranes flexible enough to function properly. Add a small handful of tasty sunflower or pumpkin seeds to your breakfast cereal, or snack on them at midday. Use sesame seeds liberally in cooking and baking—they add a subtle, nutty taste. And grind up tiny flaxseeds in a clean coffee grinder and stir into yogurt, cereal, or smoothies.

Eat with the fishes. When granny told you to eat your fish because it was brain food, she knew what she was talking about. Canned salmon, mackerel, herring, and sardines are loaded with omega-3 fatty acids. Another function of these healthy fats is that they help prevent inflammation in brain cells. Inflammation destroys cells, and when that happens in the brain it hastens cognitive decline. In a six-year study involving 4,000 Chicago residents age 65 and older, researchers found that the folks who ate the most fish were better able to preserve their memories than non-fish eaters.

Pal around with prunes. If the only time you reach for prunes is when you're a little, um, backed up, you're missing out on a marvelous opportunity to protect your memory. That's because prunes, and to a lesser extent, raisins, are superstars on the ORAC (oxygen radical absorbance capacity) chart. These tasty dried fruits are like the Terminator when it comes to neutralizing free radicals, which are unstable, cell-damaging molecules. When free radicals go on a rampage against brain cells, memory loss ensues. Have three or four prunes a day, or tuck a little box of raisins into your purse or briefcase.

Try the Popeye diet. Spinach is also way up there on the ORAC chart, and it's one of the few food sources of a-lipoic acid (ALA). This antioxidant seems to have a special affinity for protecting brain cells. In a study conducted on aging mice, researchers learned that ALA helped mice remember their way through a maze as well as mice that were much younger. Need more reasons to open a can of spinach (or enjoy it fresh or frozen) a few times a week? It's also a great source of the B vitamin folic acid, which helps neutralize a substance called homocysteine. High homocysteine levels can increase the risk for Alzheimer's disease in people over 60 by a whopping 150 percent.

When to Call THE DOCTOR

It's hard for people to assess memory problems on their own. So schedule an appointment with your doctor if you feel that your memory has slipped significantly over the last six months. And make an appointment right away (or have a loved one or a friend make one for you) if you have trouble remembering how to do things you've done many times before, can't remember how to get to a familiar place, or have trouble accomplishing activities that involve step-by-step instructions, such as following a recipe.

the natural DOCTOR'S Rx

Blueberry juice may boost your memory—aim for 16 ounces of 100 percent pure, unsweetened blueberry juice a day. And sage tea also has memory-enhancing properties. Brew a cup with 1 teaspoon of dried sage to 1 cup boiled water. Cover, steep for 10 minutes, and strain before drinking.

Crave some curry. The bright yellow spice called turmeric, used in traditional Indian curries and other dishes, gets its neon glow from an antioxidant compound called curcumin. Turmeric drew the attention of researchers who study Alzheimer's disease when they noticed that people in India, where turmeric is used liberally in cooking, have relatively low rates of the disease. And now we know why: Curcumin deters the formation of brain deposits called amyloid plaques, which are the classic sign of Alzheimer's disease. Although turmeric is part of the curry spice blend, it doesn't taste spicy hot. Its exotic, slightly citrusy flavor complements rice (and turns it a beautiful bright yellow), soups, meat loafs, stews, casseroles, and baked goods. For maximum effect, try to get at least a teaspoonful or so every day.

Seek out shiitake. In research conducted recently at UCLA, scientists discovered that the combination of vitamin D and curcumin (the key ingredient in turmeric) could help stimulate the immune system to clear amyloid plaques found in the brains of people suffering from Alzheimer's disease. Turns out, one delectable source of vitamin D is shiitake mushrooms. Although you can find them fresh in markets, dried shiitake mushrooms have a richer, more concentrated flavor.

Sprinkle on some cinnamon. Helping preserve your memory is only one reason to use this tasty cookie spice as often as possible. It reduces inflammation and is a potent antioxidant. As an added bonus, it's been proven to lower cholesterol and blood sugar. To get those benefits, as well as a potential memory boost, freely sprinkle cinnamon on sliced fruit, toast, hot or cold breakfast cereal, lattes, and even soups and stews. Aim to get ¼ to ½ teaspoon every day.

Have a spot of tea. Researchers from the Netherlands confirmed in a very recent study that two green tea components, L-theanine and caffeine, can significantly boost levels of attention and alertness. This builds on what we already knew about tea's brain benefits. In another study published in the *American Journal of Clinical Nutrition*, researchers discovered that drinking just one cup of green tea a day made folks (55 and older) 38 percent less likely to experience a decline in their mental abilities. And drinking a second cup daily made them 54 percent less likely to show mental declines.

menstrual problems

Whether you have premenstrual syndrome or just the occasional menstrual cramps, you've probably heard all the PMS jokes, and you probably don't find them very funny. Of course, bad moods and tempers are just as likely to be triggered by stress as by menstrual discomfort. But if you find yourself staring a little too long at the knife rack during *that* time of the month, these home remedies should repair your jangled nerves and ease your cramps.

first things first

What you eat can make a big difference in how you feel before and during your period. Research has shown that eating foods rich in omega-3 fatty acids, calcium, and vitamin B_6 seems to ease mood-related PMS symptoms. And eating vitamin B_1-rich foods may ease cramps.

kitchen cabinet cures

Get sunnier with seeds. Sunflower seeds are chockfull of vitamin B_1 (thiamin). In one study, 556 young women with painful periods were given 100 milligrams of vitamin B_1 or a placebo for three months. After 60 days, 55 percent of the women taking the vitamin said their pain had disappeared. In the group who took the sugar pills, 99 percent said they didn't notice any difference in their symptoms. Though researchers couldn't explain how B_1 relieves cramps, they did note that vitamin B_1 deficiencies cause decreased pain tolerance, muscle cramping, and fatigue.

Pantry HEALERS

Canned fish (salmon, sardines, mackerel, tuna)
Celery
Chamomile tea
Cinnamon
Cloves
Collard greens
Epsom salts
Fennel seeds
Ginger
Ginger tea
Lavender essential oil
Nuts
Olive oil
Seeds
Shiitake mushrooms
Spinach
Wheat germ
Whole-grain cereals

the natural
DOCTOR'S ℞

If you're among the women who get that bloated feeling before or during your period, make celery sticks your go-to snack. They're a natural diuretic and are great at helping you beat the bloat.

Moodiness is a classic PMS symptom that responds nicely to doses of sunlight—whether from Mother Nature or from full-spectrum lightbulbs. Exercise is also a perfect way to dispel bad PMS moods.

A quarter-cup serving of tasty sunflower seeds supplies more than half your daily B_1 requirement.

Feast on canned fish. Fatty fish like canned sardines, salmon, tuna, and mackerel are high in omega-3 fatty acids, which may help ease menstrual cramps. What's more, a serving of yellowfin tuna (canned as "chunk light") provides almost 60 percent of your daily requirement for vitamin B_6, which seems to improve PMS symptoms for some women.

Brew a spicy tea. Ginger tea is a cross-cultural cramp reliever, known to folk healers as well as to practitioners in America, China, India, the Middle East, and beyond. Ginger contains compounds that work very much like nonsteroidal anti-inflammatory drugs, such as ibuprofen, to suppress prostaglandins. These are the hormone-like substances that are thought to trigger menstrual cramps. Ginger also contains four antispasmodic agents that relax muscles to ease cramps. To make an anti-cramp brew, just put ½ teaspoon of powdered ginger in a cup. Fill with boiling water, cover, and steep for 5 minutes. Strain before drinking. Have a hot cup two or three times a day.

Mine your cabinets for calcium. A diet rich in calcium and vitamin D (which helps the body absorb calcium) seems to ease PMS symptoms. No one is certain exactly why this combination works—it's possible that PMS actually stems from a calcium deficiency—but it does help some women. A large study of about 3,000 women found that those who got about 1,200 milligrams of calcium and 400 IU of vitamin D from food were about a third less likely to have PMS than those who got considerably less. A serving of spinach or collard greens provides almost one-fourth of your daily calcium requirement. And dried shiitake mushrooms are an excellent source of vitamin D.

Bag some chamomile. Chamomile tea has been easing menstrual cramps for hundreds of years. The apple-scented brew has antispasmodic properties to calm cramps, and its mild sedative effects calm jangled nerves. To make a tea, pour 1 cup boiling water over two tea bags, cover, steep for 10 minutes, and enjoy two or three cups a day. Make sure to have a cup before bedtime, too—it'll help you get a great night's sleep.

Seek out magnesium-rich treats. Baked goods made with whole-grain flour, buckwheat, or whole-grain cornmeal—all rich in magnesium—could help put a stop to the PMS blues. Although it's unclear how magnesium affects PMS, the nutrient is essential for dopamine production. This mood-boosting hormone also helps balance adrenal and kidney function, which in turn helps minimize fluid retention. And in a two-month British study, women who took just 200 milligrams of magnesium daily—about the equivalent of a quarter cup of almonds or two servings of spinach—had less weight gain, bloating, and breast tenderness during the second month of the study than women taking a placebo. Another study found that the ratio of magnesium to calcium was significantly lower in women with PMS than in women without it.

Get a little nutty. Nuts, seeds, wheat germ, and other foods high in vitamin E may help relieve symptoms of PMS. In a small three-month study of 46 women with PMS, those who took a daily 400 IU dose of vitamin E—admittedly the equivalent of far more nuts than you'd want to eat in one day—saw their mental and physical symptoms of PMS abate.

Eat to beat period problems

A study of 33 healthy women found that reducing the amount of animal fat in their diets from the typical 40 percent to 20 percent made a huge difference in their PMS symptoms. Overall, their bloating, mood swings, and concentration problems lessened substantially.

Why does eating more vegetables and whole grains help women with PMS? It could be that doing so flattens the hormone roller-coaster by lowering levels of estrogen in the blood.

Another reason: Complex carbs boost levels of the feel-good neurotransmitter serotonin, the same one targeted by certain antidepressants. In a study at the Massachusetts Institute of Technology, researchers found that women who ate lots of complex carbs became less depressed, angry, and anxious and had more stable moods than women who ate fewer complex carbs.

That makes sense, because high-fiber carbs are digested more slowly than carbs that come from white sugar, flour, or rice, for example, so they help keep blood sugar levels stable. When blood sugar drops too low, fatigue and irritability ensue and magnify mood-related PMS symptoms. Complex carbs also help prevent the constipation that's common in women with menstrual cramps.

Many women admit to craving chocolate and ice cream before and during their periods. But instead of having a sugar fix, eating meals packed with whole grains, fruits, and vegetables may double-cross PMS symptoms, including the cramping that often accompanies heavy bleeding.

Find fiber in your pantry. Think of dietary fiber as a natural sponge that sops up excess estrogen. Lowering estrogen levels could mean fewer PMS symptoms. Increase your fiber intake by chowing down on whole-grain cereal or oatmeal for breakfast. Read labels and select those with the highest fiber content per serving. For an additional fiber fix, sprinkle a couple of spoonfuls of freshly ground flaxseed over your cereal (or add it to low-fat yogurt, which will also give you a symptom-reducing calcium boost).

Change your oil. Try substituting extra-virgin olive oil as often as you can for butter, margarine, and other less healthy fats. Butter is high in saturated fat, which may contribute to inflammation that exacerbates PMS symptoms. On the other hand, olive oil is rich in polyphenols, which are antioxidant substances that reduce inflammation.

Take a slow soak. Mix 30 drops of lavender essential oil with a cup of Epsom salts. Add to hot bath water and soak until the water cools. The Epsom salts will help with water retention and will ease muscular aches and pains. The fragrant oils will relax you and lift your spirits.

 ## recipe for healing

Herbal Cramp Pillow

This soothing little sack has its roots in traditional Chinese medicine. It contains spice rack herbs that are known to relieve pain.

> 2 tablespoons powdered ginger
> 2 tablespoons cloves
> 2 tablespoons ground cinnamon
> 2 tablespoons fennel seeds

1. Put the ginger, cloves, cinnamon, and fennel seeds into a bag made with several thicknesses of cheesecloth or a piece of cotton cloth. Tie securely with cotton string.
2. Put an inch or two of water in a small pot and bring to a boil.
3. Set the bag in a sieve or steamer a few inches above the boiling water and heat until the bag is comfortably hot.
4. Lie down on the couch, and place the herb bag on your lower abdomen. Relax and rest for 15 minutes or so. You can reuse the bag a few times; make a new one when the herbs lose their aroma.

motion sickness

Maybe seagoing vessels upend your equilibrium, or perhaps you can't bear to take a bus or a train. Some folks can ride for hours in the front seat of a car, but put them in the rear and they quickly turn green as grass. No matter which kind of movement provokes you, you'll find that simple kitchen remedies can help put the brakes on your distress.

first things first

Following these suggestions may help keep motion sickness in check while you're traveling.

On a plane:
- Eat low-cal snacks and light meals 24 hours before departing.
- Choose a seat toward the front of the plane or by the wing.
- Direct the air vent above your seat toward your face.

In a car:
- Sit in the front seat.
- Keep your eyes on the horizon.
- Don't read or look at maps.
- Keep your head still by resting it against the seat back.
- Turn the air vents toward your face.

On a boat:
- Ask for a cabin on the upper deck or toward the front of the ship.
- When on deck, keep your eyes fixed on the horizon or land.

Pantry HEALERS

Cloves

Ginger (candied, fresh, powdered)

Honey

Lemon

Nutmeg

Peppermint (dried)

Vegetable oil

Usually, your bout of motion sickness will end shortly after you've exited the moving vehicle or boat. Call for emergency assistance on board if lethargy, confusion, headache, stiff neck, or severe abdominal pain accompanies your nausea or vomiting. Do the same if there is a danger of dehydration (especially if the patient is a child). Symptoms of dehydration include dry lips and mouth, sunken eyes, decreased urination, and rapid pulse. Call your doctor if vomiting lasts for more than several hours in a child or a day in an adult.

kitchen cabinet cures

Pack the ginger. Without question, the most effective motion sickness remedy is ginger. The herb has been tested on people sailing in rough seas, watching dizzying visual displays, and sitting in rotating chairs. In all cases, ginger lengthened the time it took people to become nauseous and lessened their tendency to vomit.

The chemical compounds that give ginger its zingy taste—mainly gingerol and shogaol—reduce intestinal contractions, neutralize digestive acids, and quell activity in the brain's "vomiting center." But ginger is better at preventing motion sickness than stopping it. If you're susceptible, take ginger *before* you start your journey.

To use ginger, mix a pinch of powdered ginger in water or eat ½ teaspoon chopped fresh ginger every 15 minutes for one hour before traveling; continue this if any signs of illness occur. You can also drink ginger tea or nibble pieces of candied ginger before your trip.

Chew on some cloves. Cloves contain compounds that help stop spasms, so they might also relieve that sudden lurching feeling. Try grinding a few cloves between your teeth before you get into a situation that might trigger motion sickness.

Have some warm "lemon-aid." Make a warm, tummy-soothing drink by squeezing the juice of 1 lemon in a cup of water sweetened with a teaspoon of honey. Sip, as needed. Keep the drink warm in a thermos when traveling.

 ## recipe for healing

Spicy Tummy Rub

Many kids are prone to motion sickness, especially during car rides. This fragrant rub might help settle your child's tummy during your trip. Make it before you set out.

> 1 teaspoon ground ginger
> ¼ teaspoon powdered nutmeg
> 2 tablespoons dried peppermint
> ¼ cup vegetable oil

Blend the ginger, nutmeg, and peppermint in the oil, and let steep for an hour or so. Then strain. Massage the oil into your child's feet, temples, and wrists. If you're not driving, do it during car rides or on boat or plane rides.

nausea & vomiting

There's no mistaking what your body's trying to do when you're vomiting—it's ridding itself of something noxious. Nausea, on the other hand, though more subtle, is also disturbing—especially when the "am I going to throw up or not?" feeling continues for hours, or longer. Causes for the unpleasant duo are many, but most commonly the culprit is a case of stomach flu, more properly called viral gastroenteritis. Morning sickness and medications (especially chemotherapy), overindulging in alcohol, motion sickness, migraines, food poisoning, and disorders of the stomach or intestines can also throw you into a state of distress. In most cases, though, you can help your system ease up with easy remedies you already have on hand at home.

first things first

As awful as it feels to throw up, a brief bout of vomiting usually serves a purpose. It rids the body of toxic substances, and once it's over, nausea and stomach pain should cease.

Repeated vomiting, on the other hand, can lead to dehydration. To prevent that from happening:

• Drink clear liquids as soon as you can keep them down. Mint tea can be soothing.

• Wait six hours or so after your last episode of vomiting before you start eating again. Then, eat lightly: Nibble on saltines, Jell-O, and toast. Next, try bland foods, such as

Pantry HEALERS

Apple cider vinegar

Apples

Bananas

Cayenne pepper

Cereal

Chamomile tea

Cinnamon

Ginger (powdered, fresh)

Fennel seeds

Jell-O

Peppermint essential oil

Peppermint tea

Rice

Salt

Saltines

Toast

Most nausea is easy to diagnose and a short-term issue.
But if nausea and vomiting
are accompanied by these
symptoms, seek emergency
attention. It might be indicative
of a more serious health issue:

- Chest pain
- Severe abdominal cramping
  or pain
- Blurred vision
- Fainting
- Confusion
- Cold, clammy, pale skin
- High fever and stiff neck
- Fecal material or fecal odor
  in the vomit
- Severe headache
- Inability to keep food or
  liquid down for 12 hours
  (8 hours for a child)
- Vomit that contains blood,
  resembles coffee grounds,
  or is green

*Make an appointment with
your doctor if:*

- You have diarrhea or a
  temperature of 100°F
  or above.
- Bouts of nausea and vomiting have lasted longer than
  a month.
- You've had unexplained
  weight loss.

cereal, rice, and non-citrus fruit. like bananas or apples.
Avoid spicy or fatty foods.

- Give yourself a few days before you resume your normal
  diet.

kitchen cabinet cures

First, try ginger. Ginger is proven for its ability to relieve
nausea and vomiting due to morning sickness, motion
sickness, and even for the vomiting that accompanies chemotherapy treatment. In fact, a research paper published in
the *Journal of Gynecological Oncology* listed ginger treatment for chemotherapy-related nausea among the top 10
major research advances in gynecological cancer in 2009.

To prevent nausea after chemotherapy: First, talk to your
doctor and discuss taking ginger. With her OK, starting
one week before your treatment, take ½ teaspoon powdered ginger a day.

For motion sickness: Take ½ teaspoon fresh ginger or a
pinch of powdered ginger every 15 minutes for 1 hour
before traveling and continue the dose if you feel sick
during your trip.

For migraine-related nausea: Take ½ teaspoon powdered
ginger at the first sign of a migraine.

Bathe if you can't drink. If you tried taking ginger but
vomited anyway, try soaking your hands or feet in a ginger
bath. You're likely to absorb enough of the herb through
your skin to calm things down. Put a tablespoon of minced
fresh or powdered ginger in a quart of hot water in a bowl or
basin. Make sure it's not hot enough to burn you, then soak
your hands or feet in the ginger bath until your nausea subsides. Alternately, wrap the ginger in a cheesecloth bag and
float it in a bath tub of hot water and take a nice long soak.

Sip mint tea. This traditional remedy is one of the top
nausea treatments all over the world. Herbal experts
believe peppermint may reduce the gag reflex by anesthe-
tizing the stomach lining. Use a peppermint tea bag in a
cup of boiling water and cover it for 10 minutes, or make a
stronger brew this way: Put 1 tablespoon dried peppermint
or three or four tea bags in a 1-pint canning jar. Fill with
boiling water. Let stand for 30 minutes, shaking the bottle
a few times while it steeps. Then strain and sip as needed.

Have a cup of chamomile. This delicate herb contains potent anti-inflammatory and pain-relieving compounds that may ease the gag reflex. To treat nausea, put four or five chamomile tea bags (to equal about 2 tablespoons of dried chamomile flowers) in a pint jar and fill with boiling water. Steep for 30 minutes before drinking.

Crush some fennel seeds. Pleasant-tasting fennel seeds contain a compound called anethole, which has antiseptic and antispasmodic properties. Like mint and chamomile, it also contains anesthetic elements that may reduce the stomach's gag reflex. To use, buzz a tablespoon of fennel seeds in a clean coffee grinder. Put in a cup, fill with boiling water, cover and steep for 10 minutes. Strain before sipping.

Try a tummy rub. If your little one has an episode of vomiting or nausea, you can make him feel better by giving him a gentle belly rub. Mix a few drops of peppermint essential oil in a tablespoon or so of olive oil, and gently massage his belly in a clockwise direction.

Drink this for food poisoning. If you suspect food poisoning and have diarrhea in addition to nausea and vomiting, make a cup of cinnamon-ginger tea. Mix 1 teaspoon powdered cinnamon with ½ teaspoon grated fresh or powdered ginger. Add both spices to a cup of boiling water, cover, and steep for 15 minutes, then strain and sip. The cinnamon can help kill bacteria that might be causing the problem.

the natural DOCTOR'S Rx

After you've experienced a nasty bout of vomiting, your doctor will tell you to forgo dairy products until you've recovered. She's also likely to put you on the "BRAT" diet for a few days or so. That means limiting what you eat to bananas, plain rice, applesauce, and dry toast. This diet is also doctor-recommended for diarrhea.

Weird & wacky

We don't think this old folk remedy for nausea sounds very appetizing, but perhaps it worked for someone: Air-pop some popcorn and put it in a bowl. Cover with boiling water and let stand for 15 minutes. Eat a teaspoon of the soggy stuff every 15 minutes or so.

recipe for healing

Spicy Stomach Soother

This home remedy for vomiting turns up time and time again in collections of folkloric treatments. Experts suggest it might work by counter-irritating the stomach lining—think of it as fighting fire with fire.

- 1 teaspoon salt
- 1 teaspoon cayenne pepper
- ¾ cup apple cider vinegar

Mix the salt, cayenne pepper, and vinegar together in a cup or small bowl and take 1 tablespoon every 15 to 30 minutes as needed.

nosebleed

A sudden gush of blood coursing (or even trickling) down your face can really put a dent in your day, not to mention in your laundry budget. Nosebleeds can appear out of nowhere, as in when you scratch your nose and unwittingly nick a blood vessel with your nail. More often, a bloody nose results from an accidental whack while you're having fun on a sports field or court. Whatever the cause, don't panic. If you keep your wits about you, you can usually stop a nosebleed in a matter of minutes.

first things first

Some nosebleeds occur when dry air, typically during the winter, dries out nasal passages and makes them more susceptible to bleeding. That's why it's a good idea to run a humidifier while you sleep whenever the weather gets cool enough to trigger your home's heating. If you get a nosebleed, try these measures first:

• Sit straight up and lean forward to take pressure off the blood vessels in your nose and to lessen bleeding.

• With your thumb and index finger, firmly press your nostrils together and hold them closed for 5 to 10 minutes.

• Once the bleed is under control, don't pick your nose or blow it, and don't bend down for several hours. Keep your head above the level of your heart to prevent a re-bleed.

• If you do start bleeding again, blow your nose forcefully. This will clear your nose of blood clots. Then, give it a spray with a nasal product such as Afrin that contains oxymetazoline. Pinch your nose again, and call your doctor. Note: Never use Afrin for more than three days.

Pantry HEALERS

Aloe

Apple cider vinegar

Cayenne pepper

Ice pack

Olive oil

Petroleum jelly

Vitamin E

Water

Witch hazel

kitchen cabinet cures

Sniff a little cayenne. It's been called one of the best remedies for stopping bleeding, including nosebleeds. Cayenne promotes blood clotting and also acts as an analgesic to ease pain. And we have it on a pediatrician's authority that the hot stuff is an excellent remedy for a child's nosebleed, as counterintuitive as this might sound. Here's the recommendation: Put a little pinch of pepper on your open palm and let your child sniff it into his nostril. Be sure to wash your hands afterward so you don't accidentally transfer the pepper to your eyes.

Try a little witch. Dip a cotton swab in witch hazel and gently insert it into the bleeding nostril. Witch hazel is an astringent that will constrict the blood vessels inside the nose to stop the bleeding.

Apply some E. When your nose has stopped bleeding, puncture a vitamin E capsule of any dose size and squeeze out the liquid. Very gently, rub a tiny bit inside your nose to keep it moist.

Squeeze an aloe leaf. The healing, soothing, and moisturizing power of pure aloe gel is a perfect match for healing a wounded nose. Once your nose has stopped bleeding, slit open a small aloe stalk and dip a cotton swab in the gel. Very gently, apply to the inside of the nostril.

Sip some vinegar water. An old Amish trick for stopping a nosebleed calls for stirring 2 tablespoons of apple cider vinegar into a small glass of water. Fans of this remedy swear it never fails.

Put the freeze on it. Put an ice pack on the bridge of your nose or an icy cold, wet washcloth on the back of your neck for 5 minutes. The cold will shrink blood vessels and cut off the bleeding.

Drink up. Prevent future problems by keeping your mucous membranes moist. Drink eight 8-ounce glasses of water every day. Drink more if your urine is dark, which indicates that you could be dehydrated.

Lube your nostrils. On particularly dry days, dab the inside of your nostrils with a bit of petroleum jelly or even a little olive oil to keep them moist.

When to Call THE DOCTOR

Most nosebleeds are harmless. But seek emergency attention if:

• The nosebleed follows a fall, a blow to the head, or a punch in the nose. Your nose could be broken, or you might have a head injury.

• The bleeding lasts longer than 20 minutes or is very heavy.

• You have blurred vision and/or severe pain in or around one eye.

Otherwise, call your doctor if you have frequent nosebleeds, which may be linked to problems like high blood pressure, an infection, or even a tumor. Blood-thinning medications you're taking, such as aspirin or warfarin, could also be a culprit.

poison ivy/oak

So you didn't remember the famous warning: "Leaves of three, let it be." Now your skin is covered with an itchy, unsightly rash. Must you suffer in silence? The answer, happily, is no. You can walk into your pantry, pull out a few items, and whip yourself up some rash relief.

first things first

As soon as you've been in contact with poison oak, poison ivy, or sumac, take these four steps immediately. If the resin is left on your skin, it can spread to other parts of the body—and even to other people.

• Use a poison ivy wipe or wash. Formulated to remove urushiol, the toxic oil to which almost everyone is allergic, these products can whisk up to 95 percent of urushiol off the skin, studies show. Brands include Tecnu Outdoor Skin Cleanser and Cortaid Poison Ivy Care wipes.

• No special products? Try rubbing alcohol, a hand sanitizer containing alcohol, or even vodka. It will disperse the urushiol and get it off your skin.

• Rewash with soap or an ivy wash. Washing with soap will remove any urushiol that hasn't attached itself to skin proteins yet. Hopping into the shower within an hour after exposure can further cut your risk of itchy blisters.

• Urushiol is an incredibly tenacious substance and will cling to clothes and shoes. Toss your clothes into the washing machine and launder on hot with laundry soap. Scrub shoes with warm water and soap to remove all traces of the oil.

Pantry HEALERS

Ammonia

Apple cider vinegar

Baking soda

Hand sanitizer

Lavender
essential oil

Liquid shoe polish

Oatmeal

Peppermint
essential oil

Rubbing alcohol

Salt

Spray deodorant

Vodka

Witch hazel

kitchen cabinet cures

Slip into an oatmeal bath. Boil ½ to 1 pound oatmeal (not instant or flavored) in 1 to 2 gallons water for 30 minutes, then add to your bathwater. Soak in the tub for as long as you can. Commercial oatmeal bath products are also available.

Chill out with vinegar. Mix equal parts of apple cider vinegar with water, and pour into a spray bottle. Chill in the refrigerator. When you need cool relief, spritz the rash liberally with the cold tonic.

Try table salt. Many people swear that the key to poison ivy relief is to wet the skin and then coat it with table salt, with the goal of drying the rash out. Others recommend sprinkling Epsom salts into a bathtub and taking a soak.

Take a tea bath. Throw three to five tea bags into a bathtub, stir it, and then take a pleasant soak. Use black tea, not herbal. The tannic acids in the tea should help relieve the inflammation and the itching.

 recipe for healing

Anti-itch Wrap
Apple cider and witch hazel cool the burning itch, the lavender oil soothes and heals, and the baking soda neutralizes the acid that causes itch and pain.

> ¼ cup apple cider vinegar
> ¼ cup witch hazel
> 2 cups cold water
> 10 drops lavender essential oil
> 2 teaspoons baking soda

1. In a large bowl, mix the vinegar, witch hazel, and water. In a separate small bowl, mix the essential oil with the baking soda. Stir the baking soda mixture into the water mixture.

2. Soak a clean cloth in the cool solution, and wrap it over the itchy area for 20 minutes at a time or until the cloth begins to dry. Keep the solution chilled in the refrigerator for up to two weeks.

3. Repeat up to three times a day.

Generally, the weepy, blistery rash appears from two hours to 14 days after contact with the resin and lasts up to three weeks. Symptoms can include headache and fatigue. If you're in extreme discomfort, or if you have severe blistering, swelling, or redness, call your doctor. You should also alert the doctor if you might have inhaled the smoke of burning poison ivy plants, especially if you become short of breath. Seek medical attention at once if the rash is on your eyes, nose, mouth, throat, or genitals.

sinusitis

The pressure in your face feels like lots of tiny little people with jackhammers are going at it inside your head. You're stuffed up and you hurt—it actually feels like your entire face is pounding. Welcome to sinusitis, a condition that causes headache, nasal discharge, and cheekbone pain. If allergies, a cold, or the flu have left your sinuses all blocked up, handy kitchen cures can come to the rescue and provide nearly instant relief.

first things first

Before you get to home remedies, tend to the basics to help get past your sinusitis:

• Since you're coping with an infection, you need to rest. So even if the rest of your body feels fine, take it easy. This helps your body fight the infection and will hasten your recovery.

• Drink plenty of fluids—water and especially hot herbal tea. Avoid caffeine and alcohol because they can dehydrate you; alcohol can also worsen the swelling in your sinuses and nose.

• Steams and rinses, detailed in this chapter, help ease pain and facilitate drainage. If you've never done a nasal rinse, it's time to learn how. They really do make a difference.

• Keep that box of tissues nearby and use them. You want to clear out all that is being generated inside your sinuses.

• Use a couple of extra pillows under your head at night to help congestion drain and to ease sinus pain.

Pantry HEALERS

Apple cider vinegar

Baking soda

Eucalyptus essential oil

Garlic

Gingerroot

Herbal tea

Honey

Horseradish

Lemon

Peppermint

Sea salt

Thyme

Water

kitchen cabinet cures

Enjoy a horseradish canapé. This spicy-peppery root is prized for its ability to clear congested sinus passages. To use it, just stir together 1 tablespoon horseradish, 1 teaspoon olive oil, and 1 teaspoon lemon juice. Spread the blend on crackers, and nibble until you feel your sinuses start to drain. Or toss horseradish into some cooked rice or mashed potatoes, or take it straight from the spoon if you can tolerate the heat.

Make a hot ginger compress. Ginger can reduce inflammation and ease pain—these actions, combined with the heat from the wet towel, work wonders on painfully congested sinuses. Here's how: Slice up a 3-inch piece of ginger root. Boil 2 cups of water in a saucepan and add the ginger. Cover and simmer over low heat for 20 minutes. Soak a washcloth in the brew, make sure it's not too hot to burn your skin, then apply to your face for 15 minutes or so. Do this lying on the couch with your head elevated to help your sinuses drain.

Steam with antiseptic herbs. Place 3 teaspoons of dried thyme and 3 teaspoons dried peppermint (or three peppermint tea bags) in a small heatproof bowl and add boiling water. Lean over the bowl, covering your head and the bowl with a thick towel, and inhale for 10 minutes, keeping your face 8 to 10 inches above the water. Repeat two to three times a day, as needed. Thyme is antibacterial, and the menthol in mint is a natural decongestant that eases breathing.

When to call THE DOCTOR

You can usually trump most cases of sinusitis by using home remedies diligently. Call your doctor if your symptoms persist or worsen after a few days or if you have a fever over 100.5°F. See your doctor immediately or seek emergency care if you have these symptoms—they could be signs of a serious infection that needs urgent attention:

- Pain or swelling around your eyes
- A swollen forehead
- Severe headache
- Confusion
- Double vision or other visual abnormalities
- Stiff neck
- Shortness of breath

Give your nose a hand

Make like an ancient healer. Acupressure is an ancient Chinese healing art. Think of it as needle-free acupuncture. Use your left thumb and index finger to press the areas next to the inner eyes on both sides of the bridge of your nose. At the same time, use your fingers and the heel of your other hand to grab muscles on both sides of the spine at the back of your neck. Put pressure on all four points for about one minute.

Press out the pain. Weird as it may sound, giving your sinuses a finger massage will increase circulation to the area and help erase the pain. Here's how: Using your index fingers, press hard on the outer edge of your nostrils at the base of the nose. Hold for 30 seconds, release, and repeat three or four times.

Attack with eucalyptus. Eucalyptus essential oil is scientifically proven to kill several of the strains of bacteria that cause respiratory problems like sinus infections. To use, stir 5 drops of pure eucalyptus essential oil into 1 quart of boiling water in a heatproof bowl. Lean over the bowl, covering your head and the bowl with a thick towel, and inhale the steam for 10 to 15 minutes. Repeat three or four times a day while you're fighting the infection.

Sip some vinegar. Mix a teaspoon of apple cider vinegar in a glass of water and drink. This helps sinus drainage.

 recipes for healing

Lemon-Garlic Germ Killer

This natural antibiotic tea tastes way better than it sounds and is a remarkably efficient remedy for chasing away a sinus infection.

> 3 cloves garlic, peeled
> I whole lemon, scrubbed and cut into quarters
> ½ cup water
> I cup or so boiling water
> 3 tablespoons honey, more or less to taste

1. Toss the garlic, lemon pieces, and ½ cup water into a blender. Blend until the mixture is a smooth mush.
2. Pour the mixture into a clean, heatproof 16-ounce glass jar with a lid.
3. Top the mixture with boiling water; cover and steep for 5 minutes.
4. Pour the tea through a strainer into a large mug.
5. Sweeten to taste with honey and sip the entire cup. Drink this tea—which is actually pretty tasty—two or three times a day to help clear your sinus infection.

Simple Saline Spray

This easy-to-make solution clears your nasal passages and relieves pressure on the sinuses.

> ¼ teaspoon sea salt
> ¼ teaspoon baking soda
> I cup boiled water, cooled to a comfortable temperature

1. Add the salt and baking soda to the water and stir until dissolved.
2. To get the solution into your nose, use an ear bulb syringe, a neti pot, or a water pick on the lowest setting (you'll need a special adapter for this). Flush your nasal passages two or three times a day.

sore throat

Sometimes, the pain erupts out of nowhere and comes on so suddenly you don't know what hit you. Or, it can start as a little tickle that grows into a fierce, fiery feeling. Either way, a sore throat may be your first signal that you're coming down with a cold or the flu. It can make you feel just plain miserable—you can't really eat, your voice may sound froggy or disappear entirely, and you'll probably feel generally ill and run-down, depending on what's causing the problem. In most cases, all it takes to make you feel better are some soothing remedies, like those that follow. To whip them up, you'll need nothing more exotic than the healing ingredients you keep inside your pantry.

first things first

The minute you feel the slightest tingle of a sore throat coming on, do these things:

• Gargle with warm salt water (see instructions in this chapter) to help ease the pain.

• Get out the zinc lozenges—preferably ones with at least 6 milligrams of zinc gluconate. Have one every two hours. Suck on it until it's gone. Don't chew or swallow.

• Avoid kissing anyone, and don't share glasses or eating utensils. Sore throats and the viruses or bacteria that cause them are highly contagious.

• Wash your hands frequently with soap and water, for the same reason: to prevent spreading the germs to others.

Pantry HEALERS

Apple cider vinegar

Baking soda

Brown sugar

Cayenne pepper

Chamomile tea

Honey

Hot pepper sauce

Lemon

Marjoram

Peppermint tea

Pickles

Sage

Salt

Tea (green, black, or herbal)

Zinc lozenges

Home remedies can clear up
most sore throats within a
day or so. But see a doctor
if you have severe pain or
pain that lasts longer than a
week or if you have a fever
above 103°F (101°F for babies
six months or younger). If
you have strep throat, your
doctor will prescribe antibiotics to prevent serious
potential consequences, such
as rheumatic fever.

Other symptoms that need
a doctor's care include:

- Tender or swollen lymph
nodes in the neck
- Pus or white patches in
the throat
- Skin rashes with a sore
throat (could indicate
measles, meningitis, scarlet
fever, or mononucleosis)
- Ear pain

- Use a humidifier if the air in your home tends to be dry.
- Above all, don't smoke or drink alcohol while you're
sick, and stay clear of second-hand smoke.

kitchen cabinet cures

Reach for the vinegar. As soon as you feel the prickle
of a sore throat, employ germ-busting vinegar to help head
off the infection at the pass. Turns out, most germs can't
survive in the acidic environment vinegar creates. Just mix
¼ cup apple cider vinegar with ¼ cup warm water and
gargle every hour or so.

Try the all-time classic gargle. As we noted above,
the first thing most folks reach for when treating a sore
throat is salt, and with good reason. Not only is salt mildly
antiseptic, it helps dilute mucus and rinses phlegm away.
Gargle with ½ teaspoon salt in 8 ounces of warm water
three or four times daily. Some experts recommend that
alternating a salt gargle with a vinegar gargle every hour
or so will boost the germ-killing power of both treatments.

Signal a sage. This aromatic herb contains elements that
combat bacteria, viruses, and fungi. Sage is also a mild
astringent, so it relieves swollen throat tissue, and the herb
can lessen the inflammation that causes throat pain. Leading herbalists deem it an excellent gargle for sore throats.
To use, make sage tea with 1 teaspoon dried sage to 1 cup
of boiled water. Cover and steep for 15 to 20 minutes,
until it's comfortably warm. Gargle as often as necessary.

Imitate Winnie-the-Pooh. Honey has been easing sore
throats for who knows how many thousands of years. Even
the ancients recognized that honey acts as a mild antiseptic and soothes inflamed, irritated throat tissue. Here are
three ways to harness honey's healing power:

- Add 3 teaspoons honey and a squirt of lemon to 1 cup of
hot water and drink.

- Make a cup of sage tea (see above) and sweeten liberally
with honey.

- Brew green, black, or herbal tea, and add honey and a
squeeze of lemon juice.

Caution: Never give honey to babies under one year old.

Make it better with mint. Paiute medicine men and Chinese healers have something in common: Both rely on mint tea to treat sore throats. That's because mint is laced with compounds that kill inflammation, pain, and germs. In fact, this sprightly-tasting herb contains eight anesthetic compounds that can provide quick (but temporary) sore throat relief. To dull sore throat pain, make a strong peppermint tea with two tea bags to 1 cup boiled water. Cover and let cool till it's comfortably warm, then gargle until the entire cup is used up. Do not use peppermint gargle for children under the age of two.

Try marjoram. This green herb is used widely in Europe for remedying several common respiratory and infectious conditions, thanks to its antibacterial and pain-killing properties. A popular cure for sore throats and laryngitis is to gargle with marjoram tea sweetened with honey. Put 1 teaspoon of dried marjoram into 1 cup of boiled water. Let steep for 5 minutes, strain, then stir in a teaspoon of honey. Gargle as needed.

Take some heat. Add a few drops of hot pepper sauce to a cup of salt water (½ teaspoon salt) and gargle. Sounds painful, but the capsaicin in the cayenne will fool your nerve endings into forgetting about the pain. Use this several times a day for a day or two for maximum effectiveness.

Defuse pain with soda. Baking soda, that is. It's mildly antiseptic and soothing. Simply dissolve ½ teaspoon of baking soda in a glass of warm water and gargle a few times a day.

Weird & wacky

From Merry Olde England spring some mighty strange sore throat remedies. One—which was actually used widely until the 20th century—called for wrapping your own dirty socks around your throat. Our guess? Since sore throats are so contagious, and in the olden days a signal of potentially lethal diseases, the dirty socks were used to keep loved ones as far away as possible from the patient. But that's just a guess. Another English treatment involved wrapping bacon around the throat before bedtime. Finally, we couldn't resist passing along this Irish gem: To heal a sore throat, simply apply salt herring to the soles of the feet.

Blame your belly?

If you get more than your share of scratchy throats or if you have a throat irritation that doesn't abate, your problem may be related to GERD, or gastroesophageal reflux disease. When you have GERD, stomach acid backs up and can irritate your throat as well as your esophagus. One tip-off that GERD's the problem: You have no other symptoms of a viral illness. You're not feverish, congested, tired, or achy. Try avoiding foods that make you uncomfortable, and never eat right before going to bed. See your doctor if your problem persists.

Sip something sweet. Chamomile fights inflammation and even acts as a mild sedative, which comes in handy when sore throat pain puts you on edge. Make a double-strength tea by steeping four tea bags in 2 cups boiling water, covered, for 10 minutes. Gargle with half of the tea and add a little honey to the rest, then sip the tea.

Try the pickle cure. Most pickles are made either in vinegar or brine—both of which are good for sore throats. So it makes some sense that pickles or pickle juice are popular folk remedies. Many people swear by drinking a few tablespoons of warmed pickle juice, or just munching on a few pickles, as a terrific way to get temporary sore throat relief. But you might want to have food in your belly before drinking pickle juice; otherwise, the vinegar might cause some stomach distress.

 recipes for healing

Spicy Honey-Vinegar Cocktail

This concoction's ingredients kill germs, relieve pain, and soothe irritated throat tissues.

½ cup apple cider vinegar
4 tablespoons raw honey
1 teaspoon cayenne pepper
½ cup warm water

1. Blend the vinegar, honey, cayenne pepper, and water together until well mixed.

2. Take a tablespoon or two of the cocktail every three or four hours.

Sweet 'n' Salty Throat Rinse

This old-fashioned throat gargle is mildly antiseptic and very soothing.

2 heaping tablespoons brown sugar
½ teaspoon salt
¼ teaspoon baking soda
1 quart warm water

1. In a jar with a tight-fitting lid, combine the brown sugar, salt, baking soda, and warm water. Shake well before each use.

2. Gargle with up to ½ cup of this mixture as often as needed.

splinters

Almost anything can embed itself in your skin—a needle-sharp piece of wood, a sliver of glass, or a tiny shard of metal. But little slivers can cause a big hurt, especially if they lodge in a sensitive spot, such as under a fingernail. And there's always the possibility of infection if they're not removed carefully and completely. Here's how to use your kitchen pantry to minimize the damage.

first things first

Even before you get the tweezers out, if you can see that even a tiny bit of the splinter is protruding from the skin, try to remove it using a piece of tape. Just stick adhesive tape (or even duct tape) over the splinter and press down gently so the adhesive catches it. As you lift the tape, the splinter should come away with it. This works well if you have a number of tiny splinters that aren't very deeply embedded.

kitchen cabinet cures

Soak the splinter. If you've acquired a wood splinter, it might pop out on its own if you make it swell up. Add 1 tablespoon of Epsom salts to a cup of warm water, and soak the area of skin where the splinter is buried for 10 or 15 minutes. Do this twice a day. A tiny splinter might swell up so much that it comes right out, or it may swell enough so that you can grab it with tweezers.

Adhesive tape

Epsom salts

Fenugreek

Honey

Hydrogen peroxide

Olive oil

Vegetable oil

You can usually treat a splinter at home. Most of the time, they'll ease themselves out of your skin naturally. But if it's large or deeply embedded, or if it's underneath your nail or on your face, let a doctor handle it. Also call your doctor if you notice signs of infection: pain, pus, swelling, redness, warmth, or red streaks. Finally, make the call if the splinter is metal and you haven't had a tetanus shot within five years.

Try an Indian remedy. If you have an embedded splinter and some fenugreek, a spice used in making curry, you're in luck. Do this before bedtime: Buzz whole fenugreek seeds in a clean coffee grinder—you want a teaspoon or so (or use 1 teaspoon powdered fenugreek). Add just enough water to make a paste. Apply the paste to the splinter, wrap with gauze, and leave on overnight. In the morning, when you rinse away the paste, the splinter will have surfaced enough so that you can remove it with tape or just scrape it off.

Oil it up. Simply dab some olive or other vegetable oil on the area in which the splinter is embedded. It should slip out pretty easily.

Try honey. Wash the area thoroughly, apply honey over the splinter, then wrap with a clean bandage. Check every couple of hours, adding honey if needed. Many home healers swear it'll draw out the invader.

Bubble it out. Many people swear by hydrogen peroxide for getting splinters out. Just dowse the area with the peroxide; if all goes well, the splinter will "fizz" itself out. If it doesn't work, you've still cleaned the area well.

When all else fails... Make like a medic and use this doctor-approved first-aid approach. Do not try this if the splinter is embedded near the eye or on the face—in that case, see a doctor for removal.

• Wash your hands and the splinter area well with soap and water.

• Wipe a clean, sharp sewing needle with rubbing alcohol (vodka or a soap and water wash works, too).

• Break the skin over the splinter with the needle. Use the tip of the needle to carefully ease the tip of the splinter up and out.

• Now, the splinter should be easy to remove with a piece of tape or tweezers.

• Wash the spot again with soap and water.

• Apply an antibiotic ointment.

stings & bites

It's a jungle out there, and everywhere from the under-brush to under your bed lurk creatures great and small that can sting and bite—often painfully and, rarely, even lethally. Here's how to handle attacks from the various creepy crawlies it may be your misfortune to encounter. Take heart—no matter which critter left its mark on you, you'll be able to find something in your pantry to take out the sting and relieve the itch.

first things first

Start here when you or someone you love has been stung:

• If you've been stung by a honeybee, the creature will die, but she's left you something in her will—a venom sac that will spread more painful, itchy poison if you inadvertently squeeze it while trying to pull it out. Instead of yanking or tweezing, use a credit card from your wallet, a plastic knife from the kitchen, or other straight-edged object to *scrape* the stinger and sac out of the skin.

• Then wash immediately with soap and water. Your spider bite or bee sting needs to stay clean for several days to heal and avoid infection.

• Apply cold compresses. A clean cloth soaked in very cold water will temporarily relieve the pain, swelling, and itch of any insect bite. Apply it 15 minutes off and 15 minutes on. Alternatively, massage the area with an ice cube for 10 minutes.

Pantry HEALERS

Aloe

Apple cider vinegar

Baking soda

Chamomile tea

Cornstarch

Dishwashing liquid

Echinacea root tincture

Lavender essential oil

Meat tenderizer

Peppermint essential oil

Tea bag

Vanilla extract

Witch hazel

If you've been stung by a bee,
wasp, or hornet and feel faint,
have trouble breathing, have
swelling in your mouth or
throat, or a rapid pulse, call
911 and get to the emergency
room. Those are symptoms
of a potentially fatal allergic
reaction called anaphylaxis.
Also call your doctor if you
have a bull's-eye rash, muscle
aches, fever, and headache
within weeks of a tick bite
because you may have
Lyme disease.

kitchen cabinet cures

Use some bicarb. Neutralize acidic bee or fire ant
venom with that baking soda (bicarbonate of soda) you
keep with your baking supplies. Mix just enough of the
powder with very cold water to make a paste, and completely cover the bite with the paste.

Pour on the meat tenderizer. The enzyme product
you use to make tough cuts of meat chewable is an old home
remedy for insect bites and stings. How it works: The enzyme
(usually papain, from papaya, or bromelain from pineapples)
that breaks down the protein in that shoulder roast zeroes in
on the venom (which is also a protein) in the bite, reducing
inflammation and pain. Make a paste of one part tenderizer
to four parts water and place it on the bite or sting. Leave
it on for 30 minutes or less, otherwise it will irritate your
skin. (Aluminum chlorohydrate in antiperspirants—*not*
deodorants—may also help, but not quite as well.)

Head 'em off at the pass

No one wants to get stung, just like no one
wants the flu. But unlike flu germs, things that
sting are easy to see—and keep away. Here
are a few clever ways to keep bees, mosquitoes, and other similar critters away from you.

Use your baking ingredients. American
military health experts recommend combin-
ing a couple of teaspoons of ordinary vanilla
extract with a cup of water and spritzing
yourself with a spray bottle to keep mosquitoes at bay. You may love the smell, but those
little buzzers don't. Peppermint oil may also
drive them away.

Skip the spirits. Mosquitoes can sense the
lactic acid and carbon dioxide we give off from
100 feet away. And they're apparently nature's
own breathalyzers, too. Studies have found
that mosquitoes make a beeline for you when
you've consumed alcohol. So if you're enjoying
an outdoor picnic, skip the beer—unless it's
root beer.

Try the soap approach. In summer, bees are
like us—they are drawn to water to help cool
down. If you have a pool, birdbath, or other
water source that is drawing lots of bees to
your yard, do this: Mix ¼ cup of dishwashing
liquid into a quart of water, and pour the solution into an empty spray bottle. Spray any bees
that are hovering nearby. The solution will kill
the bees quickly without harmful pesticides.
Soon enough, the rest of the hive will start
avoiding your space.

Stay on the straight and narrow. Ticks love to
hide in tall grass and weeds and climb on you as
you brush by. If you're walking through a field
or the woods, make sure you're wearing long,
light-colored pants and a long-sleeved shirt so
you can spot the hitchhikers, some of which are
smaller than the period at the end of this sen-
tence. Stay toward the center of the trail—ticks
don't jump; they can only crawl on you if you
get close enough.

Mix up vinegar and cornstarch. Blend a spoonful of cornstarch with enough apple cider vinegar to make a paste and slather it over the bite. This remedy pulls fluid from the itchy bite, which decreases inflammation and the discomfort it causes. If you only have vinegar handy, swipe some all over the bitten area.

Whip on a wet tea bag. The tannic acid in tea can help reduce the swelling around a bite or sting.

Give it some mint. Peppermint essential oil can reduce the pain and swelling of a bee sting. Use a cotton swab to dab the fragrant oil on the site two or three times a day.

Witch for the itch. This is one of the best reasons for keeping witch hazel in the fridge: A few drops of this cool, astringent liquid will bring instant relief to a bug bite or sting.

Dab on some aloe vera. Snap off a stalk-like leaf of this helpful plant, slit it, scrape out the gel, and apply it directly to bites and stings to help relieve pain and inflammation.

Soak in some chamomile. Make a strong chamomile tea with two tea bags to 1 cup boiled water. Cover and steep for 15 minutes. Soak a cotton pad or towel in the tea, then place it over the bite and leave it on for 15 minutes or more.

Bugs in your ears?

If it's just a gnat or a fly, it's annoying, but if it's a yellow jacket, bee, or wasp, it can be downright scary. Here's what *not* to do: Stick your finger in your ear to dislodge the unwelcome visitor. You'll just push the bee in farther, anger it, and you'll probably get stung. Instead, use an insect's natural inclination to go to the light by standing next to a lamp or have someone shine a flashlight into your ear. With any luck, the critter will crawl out. If that doesn't work, place several drops of vegetable oil into the ear to kill the bug, then tilt your head and tug on your ear to allow it to float out.

recipe for healing

Pain-Fighting Bite Treatment

Native Americans boiled up the roots of the wild purple coneflower to treat insect bites and stings—even snakebites. Today, we know it as echinacea, the herb that helps reduce the severity of colds by killing viruses. The plant contains compounds that reduce swelling, prevent infection, and enhance healing. Here's how to use it to take the sting out of stings.

> 1 tablespoon echinacea root tincture
> 1 tablespoon water
> 10 drops lavender essential oil
> 1 tablespoon cosmetic clay

Combine the echinacea, water, and lavender, then slowly add it to the clay and blend. Apply the paste to the sting or bite. Store any remainder in an airtight container to prevent it from drying out. If you only have echinacea tincture on hand, just apply several drops of the liquid directly on the bite several times a day.

stress

You can't avoid stress. It's as natural a part of our daily lives as oxygen. And you want a little of it in your life. It can be a positive thing, a challenge that pushes you to excel, keeps you stimulated, boosts your immune system, and adds to your self-esteem and sense of mastery. But if you have a little too much of this good thing, or if stress turns your life upside down, you can be stuck cleaning up the emotional wreckage—anxiety, depression, frequent illnesses, psychological paralysis. Your body will start churning out hormones like cortisol that tell your brain and cardiovascular system that you're under siege 24/7, and that can lead to serious problems, from heart attack to stroke to chronic inflammatory diseases like arthritis. Fortunately, your kitchen cabinet is your doorway to an oasis of calm.

first things first

If a feeling of anxiousness lasts for more than a few days, make like a detective and try to figure out what's getting on your nerves. If you can't do it on your own, talk to a friend, a trusted clergyman, or a mental health professional who can look at your situation objectively and help you figure out the root of your distress.

Meanwhile, these strategies are proven to be among the best to help ease your way through turbulent times:

• Take an exercise break. You may not be able to quit your job and move to a desert island, but you can create a little oasis of calm for yourself. When you're feeling crazed, take

Pantry HEALERS

Almonds

Beans

Chamomile

Chamomile tea

Lavender
  essential oil

Oatmeal

Peanut butter

Peanuts

Raisins

Tea (green or black)

Vitamin C

Wheat germ

a walk. Studies show that taking a brisk walk, swimming laps, or doing other vigorous exercise can raise levels of feel-good chemicals called endorphins, help clear your mind, and reduce symptoms of anxiety and depression.

• Get spiritual for 15 minutes every day. Having some spiritual practices—prayer, meditation, even charity work—can help buffer the effects of most of the negatives in your life.

• Stay in touch—physically or virtually, by phone or through social Web sites or text messages—with people who make you feel good and keep you grounded. Having people in your life, studies show, can make you feel secure, happy, and able to handle life's slings and arrows.

kitchen cabinet cures

Pop a C. Make it 1,000 milligrams. A German study subjected 100 people to two of the most stressful things a human can face: public speaking and doing math problems. The group that took a vitamin C tablet had lower levels of cortisol—a hormone you produce in response to tension, fear, and anxiety—and had lower blood pressures than the group that didn't take the vitamin. The vitamin C takers also said they felt less stressed. Studies have shown the vitamin C reduces cortisol in animals subjected to repeated stress.

Have a cuppa. Even though tea contains jitter-causing caffeine, it seems to calm rather than jangle your nerves. And it may not have anything to do with chemistry. Researchers at the City University of London put 42 volunteers to the test: They asked them to fill out two scientifically validated tests that measure stress and anxiety. Then they stressed them out with a timed exercise in which they had to scan a document for the letter "d" and, based on a mark above or below it, either cross it out or pass over it. Afterward, they gave half the group a cup of tea and the other half a glass of water before repeating the tests. Both groups had equal scores before the beverages, but the tea group was far less stressed afterward: They actually experienced a 4 percent drop in anxiety while the water group had a 25 percent increase. The researchers noted that many members of the group reported they used tea to relax and, in fact, the tea group was far chattier after the test than the water group. They concluded that the tea ritual and its social aspects may be the reason it's nature's own Xanax.

Make it green. Green tea is lower in caffeine than most other teas, so you may be able to drink the five cups a day that lowered psychological stress in a large group of Japanese people in a recent study done at Sendai's Tohoku University Graduate School of Medicine. The researchers didn't identify any particular ingredient of green tea that might have been soothing, but animal studies suggest that one compound, EGCG, had both sedative and hypnotic effects that tamp down the body's production of stress chemicals.

Soothe yourself with chamomile. For people with generalized anxiety disorder, feeling stressed is a full-time condition. They constantly worry, suffer from muscle tension, irritability, fatigue, insomnia, and are sometimes easily startled. So if chamomile can help them—and a study found that taking chamomile reduced their symptoms by an astonishing 50 percent—it can certainly ease your everyday tension. Studies suggest it acts as a nerve relaxant. To make the tea, pour 1 cup of boiling water over two chamomile tea bags and let steep, covered, for 10 minutes. Enjoy the sweetly fragrant tea three times a day.

Bathe in chamomile. As you sip that tea, you can soak in the soothing scent of chamomile for a double dose of relaxation. Wrap six tea bags in a piece of cheesecloth or piece of hose, and hold it under the faucet while you fill the tub. Adding a teaspoon of lavender essential oil to your bathwater will plunge you even deeper into serenity.

Rub on a little lavender. It's one of the few essential oils that you can apply directly on your skin. Studies have found that lavender reduces stress, as measured by systolic blood pressure, which rises when you're tense. You can also shake a few drops on a tissue and carry it with you for those unexpected stressful moments that come up at work or when you're in traffic.

Grab a handful of almonds. Or any magnesium-rich food in your kitchen cabinet, including peanuts, instant fortified oatmeal, peanut butter, beans, or raisins. A study of university chemistry students found that test anxiety

Chamomile is so soothing that some recommend adding it to your bath.

caused them to lose magnesium, a trace mineral that helps relax muscles. Other studies have found that when magnesium levels are depleted, it can worsen stress symptoms. Interrupt this vicious cycle by including one or more of these foods at every meal during tough times.

Dish up some wheat germ. Along with being high in magnesium, wheat germ contains a phytonutrient called octacosanol, which may help improve your body's ability to withstand stress. Add a few spoonfuls to yogurt or cereal every day.

Have a bowl of oats. This traditional remedy is so well-accepted that a British career counseling site encourages nervous job seekers to have a bowl of porridge before they head off to interviews to keep themselves calm. Oats contain a compound called gramine, which has mild sedative properties. They're also packed with complex carbohydrates that may increase the amount of mood-lifting serotonin in your brain.

Avoid high-stress foods. Drinking coffee when you're tense is like trying to put out a house fire with lighter fluid, particularly if you're sensitive to caffeine. Alcohol may seem like a smart idea—after all, it relaxes you—but it increases your adrenal gland's production of stress hormones and interferes with your sleep. Likewise, sugar and refined carbohydrates (cake, cookies, and white bread to you) can heighten anxiety. So don't try to soothe your stress with "comfort foods" that are sweets.

the natural DOCTOR'S ℞

Do this breathing exercise to alleviate anxiety caused by stress: Breath in through your nose for 4 counts, hold your breath for 7 counts, and then breathe out through your mouth, making a whooshing sound as you do so, for 8 counts. Repeat 4 times and do the exercise twice a day.

sunburn

Think of sunburn as a bad gift that keeps on giving in all the wrong ways. Not only does it hurt and irritate you for several long days, it also causes permanent damage that can eventually lead to lines and wrinkles, liver spots, and, potentially, skin cancer. All that for a few weeks of tanned skin? Your best bet is to avoid sunburn at all costs: Slather yourself with sunscreen with an SPF factor of at least 15, and wear a hat and protective clothing when you have to be out in the sun. If you do get a burn, your best bet for relief is right in your kitchen.

first things first

When you first realize your skin has sunburn, get indoors fast and take these steps:

• Take an over-the-counter nonsteroidal anti-inflammatory such as ibuprofen (400 milligrams is about right) to block any pain and reduce inflammation.

• Either apply cool compresses, stand in a cool shower, or soak in a cool bath. This will ease the pain and inflammation of a new sunburn.

• Ignore the common advice to grease your skin up. Butter, petroleum jelly, and other greasy ointments prevent heat and sweat from escaping from your pores and are tough to remove from extra-tender skin. Likewise, ignore advice to apply ice; that can further injure already damaged skin.

• Instead, apply thinner, more natural healing ingredients like those described in this chapter.

Pantry HEALERS

Aloe

Apple cider vinegar

Baking soda

Evaporated milk

Green tea

Lavender
  essential oil

Oatmeal

Vitamin C

Vitamin E

White vinegar

kitchen cabinet cures

Snip a stalk. It's time again to use that aloe vera plant on your windowsill. You'll get that same soothing relief you get after an oven burn if you apply the aloe gel directly from the plant to your sunburn. In fact, aloe is the main ingredient in many of the pricey sunburn relief products you'll find at the pharmacy. Slit the stalk open with a knife, and scrape out the gel inside. Apply to the sunburn.

Comfort yourself with oatmeal. This breakfast staple also has skin-soothing properties and reduces inflammation. Stuff an old nylon stocking with oats and place under the faucet as you run some cool bathwater. Soak for 15 to 20 minutes and air-dry yourself, so you don't wipe off the healing oats with your towel.

Spritz on some lavender. A French chemist discovered the healing powers of lavender oil in the early 1900s. When he severely burned his hand in a lab accident and plunged it into a vat of lavender essential oil, the oil eased the pain and his burn healed quickly. Mix 1 teaspoon of pure lavender essential oil into about 2 ounces of water in a misting bottle. Shake and mist sunburned skin lightly as often as needed.

You're fried, so try some baking. Baking soda, that is. Bicarbonate of soda helps soothe skin inflammation. Toss a handful into cool bathwater and soak for 20 minutes.

Make like lettuce. Ordinary white vinegar contains acetic acid, a component of aspirin that can help relieve the pain, itching, and inflammation of sunburn. Soak paper towels with vinegar and apply like a compress to painful areas; leave them on until they dry. Be careful around the eyes, because vinegar can sting. Alternatively, pour a cup of white vinegar into tepid bathwater and soak for 20 minutes.

Got canned milk? You don't want to pull milk out of the fridge—too cold! But canned evaporated milk is just cool enough to ease the pain of your burn. Pour some on a clean cloth and apply to areas that hurt. It will provide a protein layer that will continue to soothe your discomfort.

Mix E and C. Taking 2,000 milligrams of vitamin C and 1,000 IU of vitamin E for eight days could help your sunburn heal and potentially reduce your chances for developing skin cancer in the future, say experts.

When to call THE DOCTOR

Most sunburns are first-degree burns—the least serious type—and respond well to home measures. But if your burn blisters, you develop chills or a fever, or the pain is unbearable, call your doctor. If you also have nausea or vomiting, headache, confusion, or fainting, you should go to an emergency room because you may have heat exhaustion or heat stroke.

Weird & wacky

We dug up one old folk remedy for sunburn that made instant sense—it called for having the victim bathe in an "easterly flowing stream." Naturally, the cool water would chill a burn and make the sufferer feel better. But here's one that we're sure won't soothe nearly as well: Having an elderly person "blow" the fire out of your blistered skin. (Unless, of course, it's your granny, and you're under the age of six.)

Go for green tea. Studies suggest that the antioxidant compounds in green tea help prevent sunburn and skin cancer when you apply it to skin or sip it regularly. It doesn't act as a sunblock, but it does protect skin against inflammation caused by the sun's UV rays. You need about 3 milligrams of the green tea compound EGCG per square inch of skin. One cup of brewed green tea contains 20 to 35 milligrams of EGCG, so after you sip a cup, brew a second cup, let it cool, and dab it on skin with a cotton ball after coming in out of the sun.

 ## recipes for healing

Burn-Soothing Bath

Oatmeal is known for its ability to reduce inflammation and soothe irritated skin; baking soda reduces itching and helps skin heal; and milk's protein helps ease the pain.

> 2 to 4 cups oatmeal
> 1 cup baking soda
> 1 cup evaporated (or regular) milk

1. Grind oatmeal in a food processor until fine.

2. Add oatmeal, baking soda, and milk to bathwater, or wrap dry ingredients in cheesecloth or a nylon stocking; hold under the faucet as you run bathwater. Soak for 20 minutes; don't towel dry. Caution: Do not add milk if your skin is blistered.

Aloe-Lavender Gel

This fragrant combination cools the feeling of heat on your skin, reduces swelling and inflammation, and wards off infection.

> 4 tablespoons aloe gel
> 1 teaspoon pure lavender essential oil
> 1 teaspoon apple cider vinegar
> 2 capsules vitamin E, 400 IU

1. Slit a few thick aloe stalks and scrape out enough gel to make 4 tablespoons. If you don't own an aloe plant, buy 100 percent pure aloe vera gel at the health or natural foods store.

2. In a small container, combine the aloe gel, lavender, and vinegar.

3. Pierce the vitamin E capsules with a clean needle and squeeze the contents into the other ingredients. Stir to blend.

4. Gently pat the gel on the sunburned skin. Use as often as needed to ease the discomfort. If you have large areas of sunburn, you might want to double the recipe.

toothache

Inside every tooth is an exquisitely tender nerve. A toothache is nature's way of telling you that something is rubbing that nerve the wrong way. In many cases, the problem is a cavity. Your tooth's protective outer shell—the enamel—has been eaten away by acid and bacteria, exposing the nerve underneath. Or, the problem may be a cracked tooth—chewing something hard has caused a fracture that exposes the nerve. Or it could be something else: an infection, abscess, or a lost filling or crown. While you wait to get to a dentist to fix the underlying cause, turn to your kitchen pantry to find some relief.

first things first

Take care of your teeth, and you'll never have worry about painful toothaches. The rules haven't changed much for a few decades:

• Before brushing your teeth in the morning, gargle with apple cider vinegar. It helps remove stains, whiten teeth, and kill bacteria in your mouth and gums.

• Brush and floss your teeth in the morning and at night, and if you can, after each meal. If you can't brush after a meal, drink some water, then rinse your mouth with water.

• Brush lighter and longer. Hold your toothbrush like a pencil, brush in a circular motion, and keep going for at least two minutes. Most people brush too hard and too short.

• Visit the dentist at least twice a year.

Pantry HEALERS

Apple cider vinegar

Candle wax

Cayenne pepper

Clove oil

Cloves

Ginger

Salt

Sugarless gum

Tea bag

Weird & wacky

Peanut butter and mustard for toothache? Some natural healers recommend it in an emergency. It's an edible version of a mustard plaster that eases sore muscles. In this case, you coat a chunk of peanut butter with a little powdered mustard, and stick it, mustard-side down, on the tooth. Mustard is a counter-irritant, like the capsaicin in peppers, which may interfere with pain messages your body sends to the brain. The peanut butter holds the mustard against the tooth.

kitchen cabinet cures

Apply cloves. Your grandma always kept a bottle of oil of cloves around for toothaches. It's a traditional remedy for numbing nerves, and today we know why. The primary chemical compound of this spice, made from the dried bud of an evergreen, is eugenol, a natural anesthetic. But clove oil needs to be used carefully. Pouring the oil on the aching area can actually worsen the pain if you get it on sensitive gum tissue or your tongue. To avoid that, put two drops of clove oil on a cotton ball and place it against the tooth itself until the pain recedes. In a pinch, use a pinch of powdered clove or place a whole clove on the tooth. Chew the whole clove a little to release its oil and keep it in place up to half an hour or until the pain subsides.

Mix ginger and cayenne. Mix equal parts of these two heat-packing spices with enough water to make a paste. Roll a piece of cotton into a tiny ball and stick it in the paste. Then, place the cotton ball on your tooth, carefully avoiding gums and tongue, and leave it there until the pain fades—or as long as you can stand it (the concoction is likely to burn). You can use these spices together or separately—they're both potent painkillers. Ginger and cayenne have been shown to be effective against arthritis pain, and the main chemical component of cayenne—capsaicin—has been found to help block pain messages from reaching the brain.

Plug it up. If a cracked or broken tooth or a cavity is causing your toothache, sealing it will help stop the pain until you can get to the dentist. Sugarless gum will work, as will cooled but still soft candle wax. Some traditional healers also recommend using roasted ginger to both cap the aching tooth and reduce pain. Simply bite down on the cooked ginger.

Shake some salt. A teaspoon of salt dissolved in a cup of boiling water makes a pain-killing mouthwash, which will clean away irritating debris and help reduce swelling. Swish it around for about 30 seconds before spitting it out.

Black bag it. The astringent tannins in strong black tea may help quell pain by reducing swelling. Place a wet tea bag against the affected tooth.

urinary tract infections

About half of all women will experience a urinary tract infection (UTI) over a lifetime (and women get them 10 times more often than men). UTIs start with a burning sensation when you urinate and can advance to cramps, pain during sexual intercourse, and even fever or chills. About 30 percent of all UTIs go away by themselves; others require antibiotic treatment. If you get frequent infections, use these measures to keep them at bay.

first things first

Better to prevent UTIs than to remedy them. Here are the fundamentals of prevention:

• Drink fluids, and plenty of them, every day. Keep a glass or bottle of water at your side throughout the day, and refill whenever it gets low.

• Wash your vaginal area before and after sexual intercourse and urinate immediately afterward to flush away bacteria that can be pushed up into your urethra.

• Stick with loose-fitting cotton undies and change them frequently. A warm, damp environment is more likely to foster bacterial growth.

• Change into dry clothes immediately after a swim.

• Wipe front to back. The most common cause of UTIs is *E. coli* bacteria, which dwell in feces.

Pantry HEALERS

Blueberry juice
Cranberry juice
Dried cranberries
Green tea
Rice
Vitamin C
Water

When to call
THE DOCTOR

You should always check in with your doctor for advice if you develop UTI symptoms. Call immediately if you're in a lot of pain or have a fever and chills. You may need a prescription antibiotic.

• Take showers, not bubble baths. The chemicals in bath salts and gels can irritate the urethra and make it prone to infections.

• Avoid harsh chemicals. Feminine sprays, douches, and deodorants could irritate the urethra, as can some spermicides.

kitchen cabinet cures

Drink berry juice. That popular old cure really does work: Drink three 8-ounce servings of cranberry or blueberry juice when you're experiencing symptoms for quick relief. Make sure to use pure cranberry or blueberry juice rather than juice "cocktails," which contain lots of sugar. Certain antioxidants in cranberries (and blueberries, too) alter antibiotic-resistant bacterial strains so they can't stick to the urinary tract and do their worst. These antioxidants literally cut the "ropes"—called tendrils—that anchor the bacteria to the lining of your urethra and weaken the bacteria cells themselves.

Or munch on some dried cranberries. About ⅓ cup of these dried antioxidants work like cranberry juice to help prevent UTIs, according to a small Harvard study.

Take some C. Most bacteria hate an acidic environment. One of the effects of taking vitamin C is the creation of nitric acid, which is toxic to all kinds of bad bacteria. Naturopathic doctors recommend taking 500 to 2,000 milligrams every two hours for two days, then 500 to 2,000 milligrams three times a day for as long as the infection is symptomatic. Once you've beaten the infection, take 500 to 1,000 milligrams per day to help prevent UTIs from coming back.

Microwave the rice sock. Fill an old sock with plain dry rice, tie it closed, and microwave for about two minutes. Test to make sure it's not too hot, then put the warm sock on your lower abdomen to relieve cramps or pain from a UTI.

Drink green tea. Drink two or three cups of tea daily. Green tea contains antioxidants that one recent study found can reduce bladder inflammation.

varicose veins

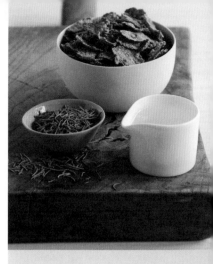

When your legs look like a road map, all you want to do is keep them covered. But varicose veins are more than a cosmetic issue: These gnarled blue veins just below the skin can throb, ache, itch, and cause blood clotting and water retention. Occasionally, they can rupture, triggering internal bleeding that can leave your legs discolored; ulcers may also form. Your doctor has myriad treatments, up to and including surgery, but try some of these home remedies first.

first things first

Our kitchen cabinet cures work, but start with these basic lifestyle adjustments to stop the situation from worsening:

• If you have varicose veins or even a family history of them, avoid prolonged standing. If you must be on your feet all day, be sure to take frequent breaks where you can sit down and elevate your legs.

• Put in 20 to 30 minutes of aerobic exercise every day. A daily walk is best since you pump blood back to your heart every time you contract your leg muscles.

• Periodically during the day, walk around to help get blood flowing. Sitting in one position too long when you have varicose veins encourages blood to pool and puts you at greater risk of a clot.

• While standing, raise yourself onto the balls of your feet and then lower your heel back down. Do this calf exercise

Pantry HEALERS

Apple cider vinegar

Bran

Canned beans

Dried blueberries

Dried cranberries

Dried strawberries

Epsom salts

High-fiber cereal

Lavender
  essential oil

Oatmeal

Olive oil

Peppermint
  essential oil

Rosemary

Rosemary
  essential oil

Witch hazel

Varicose veins tend to
worsen over time, so con-
sult your doctor when you
first notice them (they often
arrive when you're pregnant).
Call if the pain gets worse
and doesn't improve with
simple home measures or
if you develop an ulcer (an
open wound) on your leg.
Also call if your leg swells,
develops lumps, or turns red
(which could be a sign of a
clot), or if a vein ruptures
(the skin around the vein will
be bruised and discolored).
If you develop itching and a
cord-like swelling, consider it
a medical emergency: It could
be a potentially lethal pulmo-
nary embolism.

for 10 minutes several times a day to squeeze the blood
vessels in your legs to force blood upward.

• Don't cross your legs. Doing so puts pressure on your
engorged veins and prevents blood from pumping back to
the heart.

kitchen cabinet cures

Keep a fiber shelf. Move canned beans, oatmeal, bran,
and other high-fiber cereal to one shelf in the pantry and
have a few servings from it every day. Fiber will help prevent constipation, and straining can cramp blood flow and
put serious pressure on your veins.

Try the witch's brew. The astringent tannins in witch
hazel can temporarily relieve the pain of varicose veins.
Best way to use it: Refrigerate the witch hazel for extra
relief. Then soak a clean dishtowel, cheesecloth, or similar material in the chilled brew. Lie down with your legs
elevated, and drape the wet cloth over the affected area.
Leave it on until the cloth dries; repeat as often as needed.

Snack on dried berries. An antioxidant compound in
blueberries, cranberries, and strawberries seems to have
antiangiogenic properties, meaning it prevents the growth
of blood vessels. That's a vitally important quality for
fighting cancer: Preventing a tumor from developing a
blood supply will actually starve it to death. It may also
help prevent varicose veins, according to a study at Creigh-
ton University Medical Center, which looked at a product
containing berry extracts.

Sprinkle and brew rosemary. This savory herb contains a compound that strengthens blood capillaries. In
fact, that compound, called diosmin, is used synthetically in
drugs prescribed for varicose veins, hemorrhoids (varicose
veins in the anal area), and chronic venous insufficiency, a
condition in which the veins in your legs have trouble pumping blood back to the heart. To use the natural stuff, add
dried or fresh rosemary to food as frequently as you can—
it's particularly tasty in chicken, lamb, and bean dishes. You
can also get rosemary's healthy vein benefits by making a
tea. Just add a teaspoon of dried rosemary to 1 cup of boiling water. Cover and steep for 15 to 20 minutes; drink two
cups a day. Don't drink rosemary tea if you're pregnant.

Try the vinegar treatment. This folk remedy for varicose veins may require more patience and time than you're willing to give it. But at the very least, elevating your legs for 30 minutes twice a day will go a long way toward easing your vein problem. Morning and night, wrap your legs in cloths you've soaked in apple cider vinegar. Elevate your legs and rest for 30 minutes. Keep the treatments up regularly for six weeks. Some healers also recommend drinking a glass of water to which you've added a teaspoon or two of apple cider vinegar at the end of each treatment.

 recipes for healing

Healing Leg Soak

This bathtub recipe, along with the bath itself and a relaxing rest afterward, brings several proven remedies together into one wonderful treatment.

> 2 teaspoons dried rosemary
> 1 cup water
> ½ cup Epsom salts
> ½ cup witch hazel

1. Add the rosemary to the cup of water in a small saucepan; bring to a boil. Cover and steep for 20 minutes.
2. Fill the bathtub half full with hot water and add the Epsom salts and witch hazel. Filter the rosemary out of the tea and add the tea to the bathwater as well.
3. Get in the tub and soak for 15 to 20 minutes. When you get out, lie down with your legs elevated for at least 30 minutes.

Healthy Leg Rub

Rosemary helps strengthen blood capillaries, and peppermint and lavender essential oils can help ease the pain of varicose veins.

> 10 drops rosemary essential oil
> 10 drops peppermint essential oil
> 10 drops lavender pure essential oil
> 2 tablespoons olive oil

Mix the rosemary, peppermint, and lavender oils with the olive oil and gently rub the fragrant blend on your legs. Use light pressure on the veins that bulge. It's best if you elevate the legs and stroke upward toward the heart. After your rubdown, continue to rest with your legs elevated. Don't wash off the oil.

warts

They're linked in lore and old wives' tales to toads, witches, and magic, and people have used everything from snails to grasshopper spittle to get rid of them. But there's nothing whatsoever weird about warts. They're caused by common viruses—one of the 70 types known as the human papillomavirus (HPV). These can produce the little cauliflower-like sprout on the side of your finger, the painful pad on the bottom of your foot (plantar wart), and the symptomless genital condition that is the leading risk factor for cervical cancer. Your own immune system is your best defense against warts—it will vanquish 65 percent of most warts within two years, even if you do nothing. But they're unsightly, tend to spread (they're contagious!), and sometimes hurt, so it's smart to take these simple at-home measures to make them disappear—like magic.

first things first

Warts may seem strange, but that doesn't mean you need strange methods to remedy them. Start with the common-sense basics:

• Put down the scissors. Tempting though it may be to snip off an ugly wart, you're asking for trouble—pain and infection.

• Consider a store-bought wart removal product. As long as your wart isn't in a sensitive area (on the face or genitals), over-the-counter products have a good track record of successfully eradicating the problem.

• Plantar warts, which occur on the soles of your feet, can be very painful. Cut a piece of moleskin or purchase a special adhesive cushion at the drugstore to provide some padding until the wart is gone.

kitchen cabinet cures

Try a garlic patch. Garlic acts as an antiviral, but its caustic effects can potentially make warts blister and fall off naturally in a week. Just cut a peeled clove in half and rub it on the wart, cut side down. Repeat daily as needed for seven days.

Spice your food with garlic as well. Many studies have linked garlic to reduced risk of cancer—the ultimate enemy you want your immune system to fight. Why it might be effective against warts: Compounds in garlic have been shown in lab studies to fight viruses and stop them from replicating inside infected cells.

Use the banana peel trick. Some practitioners recommend taping a piece of banana peel—gooey side down—against the wart; change it daily until the wart disappears. Theories abound as to why this works: The irritation stimulates the immune system; the potassium in the banana peel helps reduce a deficiency (some believe warts are sign of a potassium shortage); the peel taped tightly to skin deprives the wart of oxygen. The truth is, no one really knows why it works, but there's considerable anecdotal evidence that it does.

Choose oats for breakfast and barley for lunch. These whole grains contain a special kind of fiber, beta-glucan, that boosts the immune system by mobilizing white blood cells and natural killer cells. There's scientific evidence that beta-glucan can even thwart tumors.

Yes, reach for the duct tape. A well-run study found that duct tape worked better than cryotherapy (freezing) on warts. Subsequent studies failed to achieve the same great results, but experts still recommend "duct tape therapy," particularly for those who are doctor- and medical-procedure–shy. Here's how to do it: Using rubber-backed duct tape (the kind used in the original study), cover the warts for six days. Then, soak the warts in warm water and rub them gently with an emery board or pumice stone. In the original study, the researchers had patients do this for as long as two

If you have genital warts, see your gynecologist; never attempt to treat these with home remedies. The virus that causes them is linked to cervical cancer.

For warts on other parts of your body, try simple remedies first, but if they don't work, make an appointment with a dermatologist. Another reason to call your dermatologist: You're over 45 and a wart suddenly appears out of nowhere. To be on the safe side, schedule a skin cancer check.

Also, have your doc take a look if a wart is red, swollen, or pus-filled—it could be an infection. If you get a lot of warts, you may have an immune system problem and should have it checked out. Finally, if you have diabetes or an immune system dysfunction, always have your physician examine any new warts.

months until the warts finally disappeared. Theoretically, the duct tape works by irritating the wart and causing the immune system to sit up, take notice, and attack it. But, in reality, no one really knows why it worked.

Add dried mushrooms to your soup. Delectable fungi such as shiitake, maitake, and morels—found in many dried mushroom mixes—contain 300 compounds, including beta-glucan, that rev up infection-fighting white blood cells.

Have a sprinkle of wheat germ. Top your morning oatmeal with this tiny, nutty part of the wheat seed, which is a powerhouse of immune-boosting nutrients, including vitamin E, the B vitamins, magnesium, potassium, iron, and zinc.

Make pumpkin muffins. Canned pumpkin is an intense source of vitamin A, which helps regulate the immune system and helps specific immune cells called lymphocytes fight off infections more effectively.

 recipe for healing

Immune-Boosting Mushroom Barley Soup

This tasty potage combines many of the pantry ingredients known to beef up your immune system—which better enables your body to fend off warts.

> 2–3 ounces packaged dried mixed mushrooms
> 2 tablespoons olive oil
> 1 cup chopped onion
> ½ cup chopped celery
> 1 cup chopped, sliced, or diced carrots
> 2 teaspoons minced garlic
> 5 cups canned low-sodium chicken broth
> ¾ cup barley
> Salt and pepper, to taste

1. To reconstitute the mushrooms, place them in a bowl and cover with boiling water (or other liquid). Allow to soak, covered, until tender. Save liquid to add to soup.

2. Place olive oil in a soup pot, add onion and celery, and sauté over medium heat until the onion is translucent, about 6 to 8 minutes. Add the carrots and mushrooms and sauté for another 6 to 8 minutes. Stir in the garlic, mushroom soaking liquid, chicken broth, and barley. Bring to a boil, then reduce heat and simmer until the barley and vegetables are tender. Season with salt and pepper to taste.

yeast infections

Yeast infections, also called candidiasis, aren't just a girl thing. Even though vaginal yeast infections are one of the top reasons women see their doctors, the fungus that causes the infection can populate your mouth (where it's called thrush), your esophagus (esophagitis), your skin, and even your bloodstream (where a yeast infection can be life threatening). It's also a common cause of a baby's diaper rash and can be passed back and forth between mother and child during breastfeeding. You'll want to see your doctor before treating any kind of yeast infection at home, but mild cases of thrush and vaginal infections do respond to natural remedies like these.

first things first

If you have a vaginal yeast infection, these simple measures will bring you a world of relief and may help prevent a recurrence.

• Go fragrance free. Perfumed powders, intimate fragrance products, soap, bath products, and even toilet paper can irritate already sensitive tissue.

• Skip the skin-tight jeans or workout outfits. Like other fungi, yeast loves a nice warm, moist environment, so you need to give yourself a little ventilation. Wear roomy cotton undies, skirts, and loose-fitting slacks if you have or are prone to yeast infections.

• Sleep naked. From the waist down, at least.

Pantry HEALERS

Cinnamon sticks

Garlic

Lavender essential oil

Salt

Tea tree oil

Vinegar

Yogurt

Vaginal infections cause a burning itch and discharge; oral thrush shows up as a white, itchy mouth rash and is sometimes the result of a depressed immune system. You should contact your doctor if:

• You're experiencing these symptoms for the first time.

• Your discharge is bloody or foul-smelling.

• You feel pain during urination or intercourse.

• Your symptoms don't go away after five days of treatment.

• You have more than three to five yeast infections a year (a diabetes symptom).

• You have discharge and a rash, especially during your period. These may signal toxic shock syndrome.

• You're pregnant.

• Your baby develops a bright red diaper rash on his bottom that doesn't clear up with the usual creams; it could be a yeast infection.

• Don't lounge around in a wet swimsuit. In fact, after removing your suit, use a hair dryer set on low to dry your vaginal area.

• Avoid hot tubs. Hot, moist…you know yeast is lurking in there.

• Eat yogurt. Studies have found that the beneficial bacteria in yogurt and other fermented milk products is effective against the yeast fungus. If you're taking antibiotics, which can destroy the good bacteria, eat yogurt containing *Lactobacillus acidophilus* or *bifidobacterium* to help replenish these *Candida* fighters.

• Avoid sugar and yeasty foods. They simply feed *Candida*, encouraging its growth.

kitchen cabinet cures

Use a warm saltwater rinse. For thrush, stir half a teaspoon of salt into a cup of warm water and swish it around in your mouth for a minute before spitting it out. For vaginal or skin infections, sprinkle a cup of sea salt into a tub of warm water and stir till dissolved. Soak for 20 minutes every day. The salt will not only speed healing, it will reduce the pain and itching.

Have some cinnamon tea. Cinnamon and yeast go great together when you're making buns, but this delicious spice has it in for yeast infections. It's a powerful antifungal that's been shown to be effective even against the nasty, drug-resistant yeast *Candida albicans*. Make a batch of tea by breaking 8 to 10 whole cinnamon sticks into 4 cups of boiling water and allowing it to simmer, covered (covering medicinal brews preserves their medicinal oils), for 15 minutes. Take the pan off the burner and allow the tea to steep, covered, for about 45 minutes. You can drink some of the tea and use the rest as a douche or to swab onto skin infections.

Try a vinegar douche. Add 2 tablespoons of vinegar to a quart of water and use as a douche twice a day for two consecutive days. The vinegar creates an inhospitable environment for the fungus. But it also makes the living difficult for beneficial bacteria, too, so don't use this home remedy for more than two days.

Eat garlic. This traditional antifungal is best eaten raw. If that sounds like something you won't relish, hide it: Chop up two cloves and sprinkle it on salads and in sauces every day. You can also mince a couple of cloves into a spoonful of honey or applesauce and swallow right off the spoon.

Treat with yogurt. Yes, eating yogurt may help prevent yeast infections. And some folk healers say that applying yogurt containing *Lactobacillus acidophilus* directly to the infection may help remedy the situation. They claim the bacteria in the yogurt produces lactic acid, which reduces the pH level in the vagina, making it less hospitable to the *Candida*. Just be sure to use plain, unsweetened yogurt, since yeast feeds on sugars. The method is simple: Dip a tampon into yogurt and insert into the vagina for 30 minutes. Repeat two or three times a day.

 ## recipe for healing

Tea Tree-Lavender Yeast Treatment
Studies have found that tea tree oil disrupts the membranes of yeast cells, and lavender kills Candida *in a test tube. Mix them together and yeast doesn't have a chance. Tea tree oil is toxic when swallowed so don't use this to treat oral infections.*

> 5 drops tea tree essential oil
> 5 drops lavender essential oil
> Distilled water

Mix the tea tree and lavender oils with a few drops of distilled water. Using a cotton swab, dab the blend on the affected parts of the body.

practical home healing

Tips and lists to help you get started

Reading practical advice makes us all feel good. There are so many positive messages: that we *can* succeed; that it doesn't take decades of experience to solve problems well; that simplicity and frugality remain valuable, viable traits. Clever advice inspires, motivates, makes us smarter. And not least of all, clever, new ideas are entertaining merely to know and share!

We hope that reading all the clever cures in this book has brought you many such feel-good moments. The question—the crucial, fundamental question—is whether you're prepared to act on the advice. And therein lies the rub. It's one thing to agree in your mind to advice; it's another thing to convince the rest of you to actually follow it.

So in this final section of *Kitchen Cures*, we want to help you take action. Not by mindless cheerleading, but rather by making it as easy as possible. Here are specific things you can do, starting the very next time you walk into your kitchen, to become an even better home healer. From what to stock in your pantry to how to store a healing concoction you just whipped up, here are resources, checklists, and tips for putting into action all the great advice you've read so far.

the healthy home pantry

You need just two things to be a successful home remedy specialist: a well-stocked pantry and a willingness to use what's stocked. In this chapter, we'll tell you exactly what items to have on hand so that you'll be prepared to act the minute you or a family member needs a healing remedy.

1 Purge the bad stuff

All the home-remedy advice in the world won't help if your pantry is packed with unhealthy food. Say it out loud: Sugary treats, processed snacks, candy, and similar products are no longer welcome here! Then grab an empty box for food to be given away and a garbage can for open packages to be tossed, and start sorting, using the following tips:

Lose the bad sugars. Sugar comes in many forms, but no matter what it's called, factory-sweetened foods should be eaten as little as possible. Though it's fine to occasionally use products that contain a little honey, maple syrup, or even white sugar for that matter, toss anything that contains corn syrup or high-fructose corn syrup within the first four ingredients. These calorie-dense, nutritionally empty sweeteners may be much worse for you than white sugar.

A shocking number of foods and drinks are thick with it, including seemingly healthy items like fruit juices, premade spaghetti sauces, and even bread. So check labels closely.

Toss the toxic fats. Get rid of anything in your pantry that lists "partially hydrogenated oil" on the label, and don't buy any products with labels listing anything partially hydrogenated. Eating these fats, called trans fats, is like putting cement in your arteries—there's no such thing as a "healthy amount" of them. These fats raise your bad (LDL) cholesterol and lower your good (HDL) cholesterol. Eating foods containing trans fats increases your risk for developing heart disease, stroke, and type 2 diabetes.

Dump products with chemical ingredients. A laundry list of chemicals means that a food product has been processed beyond recognition. Products that contain more ingredients than you can count, especially those with lots of unpronounceable chemicals, should be purged from the pantry.

Sniff your spices. If you've had that jar of thyme on your shelf for years, it's probably lost its zing—along with its medicinal properties. Take a few minutes, open each herb or spice jar, and give it the nose test. If you don't smell the herb's natural, pungent aroma when you open the bottle, it's probably lost its essential healing (and culinary) power. Toss it and replace with a fresh product. In general, most herbs, properly stored in a cool, dry, dark pantry can last a year or two. Whole spices, such as cinnamon sticks, black pepper, and whole cloves, can last a year or so longer.

Sack the loser cereals. Here's what a serving of nutritious cereal (about 1 cup) looks like. Get rid of those that fall short of these recommendations.

- 120 calories or less
- 2 grams or more protein
- 5 grams fiber (more is better)
- 8 grams (or less) sugar, unless it's an otherwise healthy cereal containing dried fruit
- 3 grams or less fat; no trans fat. If an otherwise healthy cereal contains nuts, it's fine if the fat content is a little higher.
- 10 to 25 percent of the daily value for key vitamins and minerals (e.g., iron, folate, B_6, and B_{12}).

Check for expiration dates. Though not all outdated pantry items are unhealthy, there's a good chance they've lost their nutritional value and should be discarded.

Banish sugary drinks. If you could do just one thing to improve your family's health, strictly limiting their intake of sugary drinks, including sodas and fruity drinks, would be it. That's because these beverages are the number one source of added sugars in the typical Western diet, according to a recently issued scientific statement from the American Heart Association. In America, the typical adult consumes a whopping 29.8 teaspoons of sugar a day, nearly half of which comes from soda and sweetened beverages.

The report links drinking these to a higher body weight and lower intake of essential nutrients—not to mention metabolic abnormalities (think diabetes) and a destructive impact on heart health, among other concerns.

Get wise to "natural." Some food marketers list terms like "natural" or "healthy" on product labels. That's meaningless, because there are no standards governing the use of the word. If you're interested in "natural" products, skip the promotional messages and read the nutrition label to make sure the product is free of chemical ingredients.

Organize, then shop

It may sound obvious, but when you shop with a list organized by the layout of your store, it speeds and simplifies your trip. A list also helps you resist impulse purchases that jack up your bill (and may be less nutritious than what's on your list).

If you can, avoid shopping with little kids, especially when you're in a hurry. Colorfully packaged cereals and junk foods are designed to inspire desire in children, and it can be hard to resist your kids' pleas. Take them along only when you have plenty of time and energy. Make sure they're well-fed and rested, and use the opportunity to teach them about reading labels and selecting healthy products over less nutritious ones.

You, too, should be well-fed before you shop. Walking through the grocery store when you're starving makes you want to buy everything in sight. If you don't have time to eat a full meal, at least munch an apple and drink a large glass of water before heading into the store.

2 Stock the good stuff

Once you've gone through the pantry and tossed out the stuff that's not so good for you and your family, check to see which of these items you already have on your shelves. Then shop as needed for the staples you'll want to have on hand to make home remedies—and healthful meals—for your family. For a truly healthy pantry, you should have many of the following ingredients.

Canned or dry legumes and vegetables

Beans: cannellini, kidney, chickpeas (garbanzos), pinto, black, and other varieties
Carrots
Corn
Leafy greens such as spinach and collards
Lentils
Sauerkraut
Split peas
Tomatoes, whole, crushed, pureed

Cereals and whole grains

Bulgur
Cereal, high-fiber, low-sugar
Barley, regular and quick-cooking
Oat bran
Oats, rolled and steel-cut
Quinoa
Wheat bran, unprocessed
Wheat germ
Whole-wheat couscous
Whole-wheat flour
Whole-wheat pasta

Condiments

Capers
Horseradish
Hot pepper sauce
Mustard
Sea salt
Salsa
Tamari or soy sauce

Dried fruit

Apricots
Blueberries
Cherries
Cranberries
Dates
Figs
Prunes
Raisins

Fish (canned)

Anchovies
Caviar, red and black (salmon and lumpfish)
Chunk light tuna
Herring
Sardines, packed in sardine oil
Wild Alaskan salmon
Mackerel

Groceries

Baking soda
Borax
Broth, low-sodium, preferably organic (available in cans or cartons): chicken, vegetable, and beef
Brown sugar
Chocolate, dark (65 percent cacao or higher)
Coffee
Cocoa powder
Cornstarch
Lemons
Limes
Mushrooms, dried
Onions
Granulated sugar
Plastic storage bags, assorted sizes
Tea bags: black, chamomile, green, peppermint, rooibus

Health food and drug store items

Almond oil
Avocado oil
Beeswax
Cosmetic clay
Epsom salts
Essential oils (see pages 244–246)
Honey, flavored and raw (health food stores typically offer more varieties than supermarkets)
Jojoba oil
Rubbing alcohol
Vegetable glycerin
Witch hazel

Herbs and spices

Aloe plant, potted (for your windowsill)
Black pepper
Caraway seeds
Cayenne pepper, ground
Cinnamon, ground
Cloves, whole
Coriander, ground
Cumin
Dill seed
Fennel seed

Fenugreek seed
Garlic, fresh
Ginger: fresh root, powdered root, crystallized slices
Horseradish
Lemon balm plant, potted (windowsill or garden)
Mint plant, potted (windowsill or garden)
Mustard (powder, such as Coleman's)
Mustard seed, brown or yellow
Nutmeg
Oregano
Peppermint
Rosemary
Sage
Thyme
Turmeric, ground
Wasabi

Juices

Blueberry juice (100 percent pure, unsweetened)
Cranberry (100 percent pure, unsweetened)
Grape (100 percent pure, unsweetened)
Tomato juice, low-sodium
Vegetable cocktail (100 percent vegetable juice, no sugar, low-sodium)

Oils and shortenings

Canola oil
Grapeseed oil (subs in recipes for olive oil, good for high-temperature cooking)
Virgin olive oil (use for cooking)
Extra-virgin olive oil (Look for the words "cold-pressed" on the label for the best quality; use for dressings.)
Toasted sesame oil and light sesame oil
Walnut oil (nice for salads)
Flaxseed oil (Buy refrigerated oils from good health or natural food stores and keep refrigerated. Never heat. Use it frequently because it's highly perishable. Discard if it develops an off odor.)

Nuts and seeds

Almonds
Brazil nuts
Flaxseeds
Pecans
Pistachios
Sesame seeds
Sunflower seeds
Walnuts

Vinegar

Apple cider vinegar
Distilled white vinegar
Wine vinegar

Spirits (optional)

Dark rum
Red wine
Vodka

Storage tip for nuts

Nuts and seeds spoil quickly. Store them in airtight containers and use within a month or two. Flaxseeds have an especially short shelf life. If nuts lose their nutty flavor or have an off taste, discard them and replenish your supply with fresh nuts.

the healthy shopper

Having a shopping list is a huge help in making your grocery choices smarter and healthier, and we hope the pantry guide on the previous pages helps you organize your needs. To go the next step, here are tips for knowing what to do when standing in the grocery aisle, staring at a bewildering array of seemingly similar products.

1 Shop for fresh foods first, not last.

That usually means starting in the produce section and working your way around the perimeter of the store to buy meats, seafood, dairy and fresh baked goods. Only when you've picked up all your perishable goods should you dip into the aisles for the canned and boxed foods you need to fill your pantry and round out your meals. Make this a habit, and you'll find that your cart increasingly contains healthy foods in their more natural state.

2 Choose brown grains, not white.

This holds true for products in several aisles of the grocery store: pasta, bread, crackers, rice, flour, and even the cooking-grains section. Here's why: When grains are processed and milled (giving them their white color), the most nutritious parts are stripped away. For example, when whole-wheat grain is milled into white flour, the grain's germ and bran are discarded. The germ contains concentrated nutrients; the bran, the grain's outer "skin," contains most of the grain's fiber. A similar process removes the bran and germ from rice grains to produce white rice, making brown rice the more nutritious choice.

Look for whole-grain pastas and couscous, mixes that contain barley, instant brown rice, and even whole-grain crackers. Other excellent whole grains include barley, buckwheat, bulgur, oatmeal, wild rice, and popcorn.

3 Choose brown sweeteners, not white.

By white sweetener, we mean refined sugar. By brown, we mean honey, maple syrup, and agave nectar. Now, we have to be honest: In terms of nutrition, *no* sweetener is all that good for you. But refined sugar is definitely the worst—it metabolizes extremely fast, causing fast blood-sugar surges that are bad for your health in so many ways. Plus refined sugar has no useful nutrients; it's pure, empty calories. And oddly enough, sugar isn't all that sweet—you need a lot of it in comparison with some other sweeteners. In contrast, honey, maple syrup and agave nectar all are straight from nature, and so contain far more minerals and nutrients than sugar. Plus, they are often sweeter in flavor, so you need less in your food or drink. If you wish to go the artificial sweetener route, we recommend two: xylitol and stevia. They are the healthiest, and have far less effect on blood sugar than other sweeteners.

4 Take your time in the bread section.

It's tricky, because there's little correlation between the color of the bread and what's in it. Some brown-colored "wheat" breads are made from refined flour, but colored with molasses; some whitish breads are made from whole wheat. What to do: Pick only breads in which "whole grain" is listed as the first ingredient—whole wheat, white whole wheat, whole oats or rye, for example. Also look for 3 grams of fiber or more per serving. If the first ingredient on the list is simply "wheat flour," then it's made from the same wheat as white bread—which means, stripped of fiber and nutrients.

5 Pick the right olive oil.

You want two types in your kitchen: a large container of virgin olive oil for cooking, and a small bottle of a high-quality extra-virgin olive oil for dressings and medicinal recipes.

6 Choose prepared foods with short ingredient lists.

You don't have to cut out prepared foods entirely. Just remember: The fewer and more natural-sounding the ingredients are, the healthier the food usually is. Of course, if the top ingredients are sugar and butter, put the item back on the shelf. And watch the sodium content: Even otherwise healthy processed foods can contain a day's worth of sodium. Avoid products that have more than 500 milligrams of sodium per serving.

7 Stock dried mushrooms.

Delectable dried mushrooms make a scrumptious, meaty addition to soups, stews, sauces, and egg dishes. They keep forever on your pantry shelf and offer a surprising powerhouse of benefits, depending on the species. Generally speaking, mushrooms are excellent sources of vitamin D, B vitamins, selenium, and tryptophan. Many contain compounds that help protect you against viral infections, and some mushrooms even appear to have anticancer actions. Look for dried mushroom blends that combine a few varieties—shiitake, maitake, oyster, crimini, button, portabella, and morels—to get the most nutritional bang for your buck.

8 Buy healthy add-ins for plain cereals.

Fiber-rich cereals such as bran flakes can, frankly, be a little boring. The best breakfast-cereal strategy is to buy unsweetened cereals and then add in your favorite flavors. That helps you bypass all the empty sugary calories—and lets you enjoy the cereal more. For ease, keep a wide-mouth, well-sealed jar on your counter with shelf-stable ingredients for quick mix-ins. Keep a scoop and ziplock bags handy, and you've got a handy, nutritious meal or snack for home or on the go. Stock these wise pantry shelf add-ins:

- Raisins
- Dried berries
- Almond slivers
- Pumpkin seeds
- Walnuts

the home remedy chef

If you can make a salad dressing, you can make a skin cream or cough remedy. It doesn't take any special skill or know-how to make home remedies that really work. But just like making a cake, you don't want to stray from the recipes. Here's some additional guidance for remedy-making success.

Have the right tools

The basic gear. As with cooking, there's more to making home remedies than just having the ingredients. Here's a comprehensive list of the equipment you would use if you were to make all the remedies in this book:

- Glass, stainless steel, or enameled double boiler
- Set of nonreactive mixing bowls
- Stainless steel or ceramic funnel
- Stainless steel measuring and stirring spoons
- Wooden stirring and mashing spoons
- Stainless steel, glass, or ceramic lemon squeezer or reamer
- Tea kettle
- Ceramic tea bowls and cups
- Tea strainer
- Kitchen knives
- Coffee or spice grinder, reserved for home remedy use
- Blender
- Large plastic basin, for soaking feet
- Large bowl, for facial steams
- Neti pot for sinus rinsing, available at health food stores
- Grater, reserved for grating beeswax (it's almost impossible to clean wax from a grater)
- Cheesecloth for making poultices and bath "tea bags"
- An Ace bandage or two, for holding poultices in place
- Supply of pint and quart canning jars
- Aromatherapy diffuser, available at health food stores

Choose nonreactive equipment. This will protect your health and beauty preparations from chemical reactions that can affect the color and fragrance of your remedies. That means avoiding uncoated aluminum, iron, or copper cookware.

Yes, they can serve double duty. Most of the equipment mentioned above might already be in your kitchen. Yes, you can use the same stuff for cooking as you do making home remedies. Just be sure that everything has been cleaned very well and is completely dry before starting.

Remedy making and storing advice

Select safe storage jars and dispensers. Look for small opaque jars with wide mouths and tight-fitting lids for storing your beauty creams or skin ointments. Because your home remedies don't contain preservatives, they need to be kept away from light and air. Any tinted or colored glass—amber, white, or blue—protects creams from light. Keeping a cream in a small container that it fills almost completely also protects it from air. In fact, when you use up half a jar of cream, decant the remaining cream into a smaller jar to protect it further. Tight-fitting lids are important to keep out air and prevent evaporation. Cork lids are too porous to be safe.

Also be on the lookout for spray bottles and pint-size bottles with tight lids for mouthwashes and spritzes you'll be making. You can probably recycle these from your regular kitchen and bathroom supplies. Before using storage jars, sterilize them in the dishwasher or scrub them well with soap and hot water, rinse thoroughly, and let them air-dry.

Work on a protected surface. While none of the ingredients in home-remedy recipes is all that strong, some could discolor or harm certain countertop materials. For this reason, we recommend creating your remedies on a large, washable cutting board. Choose boards made from high-density polypropylene, which is antimicrobial, nonporous, and nonabsorbent. Only work on it when it's completely dry.

Put bottle tops back on right away! You don't want bottles of hydrogen peroxide, rubbing alcohol, or essential oils left unopen in a work area. First, they evaporate fast. Second, they spill. The moment you've poured out what you need, put the top back on, tightly.

Be a wise hoarder. Most of the home remedy recipes in this book are for products that are intended to be used immediately or within a few days, so if you store a remedy at all, the safest place is in the refrigerator. You can keep some ointments and other remedies for longer; each recipe will advise you.

Don't forget the label! If you are making one of the recipes that can be safely stored, be sure to label each new jar or bottle as soon as you fill it. The label should give the product's name and the date on which it was prepared. If you're planning to give a homemade beauty product as a gift, list its ingredients as well (you don't want to inadvertently cause an allergic reaction). Labeling is crucial, because many of these preparations look alike in the bottle, and it's easy to forget what you made and when.

Use a permanent marker. When making labels, use a permanent waterproof marker, and consider covering the label with clear package tape. This will keep labels from smearing and becoming illegible—especially good for potions that contain oil.

Make tea ice cubes. Next time you brew up a strong medicinal tea, especially one that you're likely to use frequently, triple or even quadruple the recipe. Use what you need now, then let the rest cool to room temperature. Pour the tea into ice cube trays or single-serving containers, label clearly with the tea name and date, then freeze. Once the cubes are frozen, you can pop them into a freezer bag (don't forget to label it, too) for easier storage. Next time you need some tea, open your freezer and heat it up. Tip: Calming lemon balm tea ice cubes are extra-refreshing to use in regular iced tea.

a greener, cleaner home

If you think it's rewarding to make your own home remedies, just wait until you start whipping up your own home cleaning products. You'll be impressed with how effectively these simple formulas—several of which use healing ingredients mentioned throughout this book—remove dirt and kill germs. And you'll be tickled to see how much money you'll save in the process. Here's another thing that will make you smile: You won't be polluting your indoor atmosphere with potentially harmful chemicals, and you won't be exposing your family to the toxins found in many commercial cleaning products.

The five magic ingredients

You've read about these ingredients (with the exception of borax) elsewhere in this book, and here, you'll discover that they do double duty as simple home cleansers. How do we know they work? Simple: They've cleaned untold millions of homes over the decades, particularly in the days before fancy, chemical commercial cleaners ever graced store shelves. Plus, there's science to support them: Their chemical properties and pH levels (that is, alkalinity or acidity) neutralize germs and break down grease and dirt. With these five simple ingredients, you can safely clean and shine pretty much your entire home.

• Baking soda
• Borax
• Lemon juice
• White vinegar
• Tea tree essential oil

Borax, the one ingredient on the list that isn't detailed elsewhere in this book, is a natural mineral made of sodium, boron, oxygen, and water. It has properties that make it a terrific natural cleanser. It disinfects and acts as a natural laundry booster, fungicide, and multipurpose cleaner. Don't mistake borax for boric acid, by the way—they are different and not interchangeable.

Though borax is natural, it's not entirely without risks—like many natural substances, it can be toxic if ingested. Store it out of children's reach, don't use it around food, and just to be on the extra safe side, use borax in a well-ventilated area or wear a face mask when cleaning with it.

As for making the recipes below, this helpful note: The amounts are flexible. Since every cleaning situation is different, you may need to use a little more or a little less of a particular ingredient to get the job done.

recipes for home cleaning

All-Purpose Surface Cleaner

1 teaspoon borax
½ cup white vinegar
3 tablespoons fresh lemon juice
1½ cups water

Add the borax, vinegar, lemon, and water to a bowl and stir well until the borax is completely dissolved. Use a funnel to pour the solution into a spray bottle and use freely to clean kitchen surfaces. If you double or triple the recipe, you can also use this to mop kitchen and bathroom floors. In all cases, rinse thoroughly.

No-Scratch Pot Scrubber

¼ cup baking soda
White vinegar

Put the baking soda in a bowl, and add just enough white vinegar to make a thick, spreadable paste. (When you add the vinegar to the baking soda, the mixture will bubble.) Use with a plastic scrubbing sponge to clean pots and pans; the mixture won't scratch no-stick finishes.

Glass Cleaner

1 cup water
1 cup white vinegar

Combine the water and vinegar in a spray bottle and use to clean and shine any glass surface. To make the glass extra-shiny, use newspaper instead of paper towels.

Bathroom Tile Mold-and-Mildew Spray

¼ cup borax
2 cups hot water
¼ teaspoon tea tree essential oil
5 to 10 drops thyme essential oil

Stir the borax into the hot water in a bowl until it's completely dissolved. Add the tea tree and thyme essential oils and pour the mixture into a spray bottle. Spritz on the mold-darkened grout and scrub with a stiff brush. Depending on how badly the grout is mildewed and how long you've had the problem, you may need to use some elbow grease and repeat the treatment a couple of times. Once you've gotten rid of the mold, spray the solution on the tiles after every shower to keep mildew at bay. Note: The borax may make the tub or shower slippery, so rinse the surfaces thoroughly and be careful getting in and out.

all about essential oils

Essential oils capture both the fragrance and complex healing chemicals contained in certain medicinal plants. Here's what you need to know about them. When inhaled, these concentrated essences pass directly to nerve centers in our brain, where they produce a wide range of responses. Essential oils can help relieve anxiety and depression, tame our physical reactions to stress, induce sleep, and enhance energy. Research shows that the scents of certain herbs—such as lavender, bergamot, marjoram, and sandalwood—actually alter brain waves, helping to induce relaxation and sleep. When used topically or in steam inhalations, essential oils help ease pain, clear up skin problems, relieve congestion, and treat fungal, viral, and bacterial infections.

Though the word "oil" is part of their name, essential oils are very different than oils you use for cooking. Cooking oils, like olive or canola oil, come mostly from seeds or nuts. But essential oils are highly concentrated volatile distillations of leaves and flowers. They vaporize easily, and they don't leave a greasy stain like cooking oils do. In fact, they don't even feel oily. They are called "essential" because they capture most of the chemical compounds that give a plant its unique fragrant and medicinal qualities.

Because essential oils are highly concentrated, you must dilute them in a "carrier oil," such as olive, almond, sesame, or jojoba oil, before you can apply them to your skin. One notable exception is lavender essential oil, which is gentle enough to be directly applied.

Though essential oils are expensive, most recipes in this book call for just a few drops. Most of the essential oils we recommend will cost under $20 for a bottle that should last you a year or two, depending on how often you use it.

Shopping and storage tips

To make sure you purchase high-quality 100 percent pure essential oils, buy them at a reputable health food store or online.

Many essential oils can be stored for years without losing their potency. Keep them in dark bottles, tightly sealed, preferably in a cool place and always away from sunlight. Never consume essential oils; most are toxic when ingested. Store them securely, and keep them well out of children's reach.

If you're interested in exploring aromatherapy—the healing art of using aromas to stimulate health—consider consulting an aromatherapist for guidance. You should be able to find a qualified practitioner at a good local day spa. Be sure she has a state license to perform the services she offers, such as massage or beauty services. As of yet, no states have a licensure process for aromatherapists.

20 top healing oils

1 Basil
Latin name: *Ocimum basilicum*
Properties: Antiseptic, eases muscle spasms, expels digestive gas, calms nerves, eases PMS symptoms
Uses: **Headaches, bronchitis, colds, coughs, cosmetic applications**
Cautions: Avoid during pregnancy

2 Bergamot
Latin name: *Citrus bergamia*
Properties: Pain reliever, antibacterial, eases muscle cramps, deodorant, antidepressant
Uses: **Eczema, depression, anxiety, acne, bad breath, colds, bronchitis, insect repellent**
Cautions: Don't use on skin exposed to sun; may irritate sensitive skin

3 Chamomile
Latin name: *Anthemis nobilis*
Properties: Pain reliever, antidepressant, anti-inflammatory, antiseptic, sedative
Uses: **Skin problems, stress, arthritis, bursitis, blisters, wounds, menopause, PMS**
Cautions: Avoid in first trimester of pregnancy

4 Clove bud
Latin name: *Syzygium aromaticum*
Properties: Pain reliever, especially for oral problems
Uses: **Tooth pain, gum problems**
Cautions: Avoid during pregnancy

5 Cypress
Latin name: *Cupressus sempervirens*
Properties: Antiseptic, eases muscle spasms, astringent, deodorant, decongestant
Uses: **Asthma, coughs, bruises, sinusitis, insect repellent, stress**
Cautions: Avoid during pregnancy or if you have high blood pressure

6 Eucalyptus
Latin name: *Eucalyptus globulus*
Properties: Pain reliever, decongestant, expectorant, antiviral, antibacterial, antifungal
Uses: **Asthma, coughs, bronchitis, arthritis, headache, wounds, fever, insect repellent**
Cautions: Dilute before using on skin; avoid if you have epilepsy or high blood pressure

7 Fir, White
Latin name: *Abies alba*
Properties: Antiseptic, anti-inflammatory, expectorant
Uses: **Coughs, colds, muscle aches**
Cautions: Do not use on skin if bottle has been stored over one year

8 Geranium
Latin name: *Pelargonium graveolens*
Properties: Pain reliever, anti-inflammatory, antiseptic, antidepressant, deodorant, insect repellent
Uses: **Menopause, menstrual problems, breast tenderness, stress, PMS, anxiety**
Cautions: Avoid in early pregnancy; overuse may cause insomnia

9 Ginger
Latin name: *Zingiber officinale*
Properties: Antiseptic, relieves muscle spasms, expels digestive gas, pain reliever, anti-inflammatory
Uses: **Congestion, coughs, colds, headaches, fever, arthritis, nausea**
Cautions: May irritate sensitive skin

10 Grapefruit
Latin name: Citrus paradisi
Properties: Antidepressant, antiseptic, astringent
Uses: **Acne, oily skin, muscle stiffness, headache, stress, fatigue**
Cautions: Don't expose treated skin to sun

11 Lavender
Latin name: Lavendula officinalis, L. angustifolia
Properties: Antiseptic, antidepressant, antiviral, sedative, relieves muscle spasms, astringent
Uses: **Skin problems, arthritis, pain, gout, stress, anxiety, insomnia**
Cautions: Avoid if you have extremely low blood pressure

12 Lemon
Latin name: Citrus limonum
Properties: Antiseptic, eases muscle spasms, astringent, kills bacteria, antifungal, insect repellent, antiviral
Uses: **Acne, boils, exfoliant, oily skin, fever, PMS, painful joints, depression, fatigue**
Cautions: Don't expose treated skin to sun; may irritate sensitive skin

13 Lemon balm
Latin name: (Melissa) *Melissa officinalis*
Properties: Antiviral (effective against herpes); antifungal, relieves muscle spasms, sedative
Uses: **Cold sores, depression, stress, athlete's foot**
Cautions: Lemon balm is expensive to produce; bargain brands may be blended with cheaper oils

14 Myrrh
Latin name: Commiphora myrrha
Properties: Anti-inflammatory, antifungal, kills germs, astringent, expectorant
Uses: **Wounds, athlete's foot, mouth ulcers, sore throat, gum problems, laryngitis**
Cautions: Avoid during pregnancy

15 Peppermint
Latin name: Mentha piperita
Properties: Pain reliever, antiseptic, relieves muscle spasms, astringent, expels digestive gas, eases stomach pain, decongestant, antifungal
Uses: **Headache, fever, colds, sinusitis, nausea, muscle spasms, ringworm, bad breath, lethargy, depression**

Cautions: May irritate skin; do not use on damaged or broken skin

16 Rosemary
Latin name: Rosmarinus officinalis
Properties: Pain reliever, antiseptic, eases muscle spasms, decongestant, stimulant
Uses: **Fatigue, asthma, bronchitis, cramps, muscle soreness, arthritis, headache, memory booster, oily hair, dandruff, stress, depression**
Cautions: Avoid if you have high blood pressure or a history of epilepsy; do not use on broken or damaged skin

17 Sage, Clary
Latin name: Salvia sclarea
Properties: Antidepressant, deodorant, relaxes cramps
Uses: **PMS and menopause symptoms, skin toner, acne, dandruff, depression, stress, migraine, fatigue**
Cautions: Do not confuse with garden sage (*Salvia officinalis*); overuse may cause headaches

18 Tea tree
Latin name: Melaleuca alternifolia
Properties: Antibiotic, antibacterial, antiviral, decongestant
Uses: **Cuts, abrasions, insect bites, mouth ulcers, cold sores, herpes, chicken pox, colds, bronchitis, acne, athlete's foot, nail fungus, ringworm, dandruff**
Cautions: Possible irritant to sensitive skin

19 Thyme
Latin name: Thymus vulgaris
Properties: Antibacterial, pain reliever
Uses: **Arthritis, skin problems, wounds, acne, colds, sinus infections**
Cautions: Avoid red thyme oils; thyme essential oil should be a pale yellow color

20 Ylang-ylang
Latin name: Cananga odorata
Properties: Antiseptic, antidepressant, sedative
Uses: **Anxiety, stress, acne, insomnia, depression, PMS**
Cautions: Avoid use on damaged or sensitive skin

index